T0383746

Learning the Hard Way in Clinical Internships in Social Work and Psychology

In this book, Susan A. Lord shares important stories and lessons from two undergraduate and two postgraduate clinical internships as colorful narratives that will augment texts in undergraduate and graduate practicum seminar classes. The chapters engage with fundamental issues, including the importance of safety and relationship-building, good supervision, the complexities of situationally determining what constitutes ethical practice, boundary-setting, suicide assessment, and professional identity development. Narratives about making mistakes, or "learning the hard way", include being robbed at gunpoint in Chicago, being stalked by a client, and sexual harassment.

Each chapter concludes with a list of reflection, small group discussion, and class discussion questions designed to help the reader more deeply engage with the material on a personal, academic, and professional level. Written for students who are excited to begin their practicum experiences, this book explores how these experiences might be addressed and crucially stresses the importance of remembering that everyone is human and that clients are well-defended and resilient. A valuable resource for learning about the importance of safety, boundaries, and relationship development in any internship or practicum experience, it will appeal to students and scholars with interests in psychoanalysis, internship education, and relational psychotherapy.

Susan A. Lord is Clinical Associate Professor Emerita at the University of New Hampshire, USA.

Explorations in Mental Health

For more information about this series, please visit www.routledge.com/
Explorations-in-Mental-Health/book-series/EXMH

Learning the Hard Way in Clinical Internships in Social Work and Psychology

Lessons for Safety, Boundary-Setting, and Deepening the Practicum Experience

Susan A. Lord

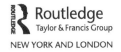

Routledge
Taylor & Francis Group

NEW YORK AND LONDON

First published 2024
by Routledge
605 Third Avenue, New York, NY 10158

and by Routledge
4 Park Square, Milton Park, Abingdon, Oxon, OX14 4RN

Routledge is an imprint of the Taylor & Francis Group, an informa business

Disclaimer: the names of all parties involved, aside from the author and unless otherwise indicated, have been changed to protect privacy and confidentiality.

Trademark notice: Product or corporate names may be trademarks or registered trademarks, and are used only for identification and explanation without intent to infringe.

ISBN: 978-1-032-59064-6 (hbk)
ISBN: 978-1-032-59198-8 (pbk)
ISBN: 978-1-003-45347-5 (ebk)

DOI: 10.4324/9781003453475

Typeset in Times New Roman
by Apex CoVantage, LLC

To all of the students, teachers, supervisees, supervisors, colleagues and, most importantly, clients that I have had the privilege of learning from and collaborating with over the years.

Contents

Introduction

My students often told me that I should write a book based on the stories I told as I was teaching. Many of these stories came from experiences of learning "the hard way" during my undergraduate and graduate practicum internships in social work and psychology. They offered some vivid and memorable illustrations of the many "mistakes" I made along the way, along with a few "successes".

I have always believed that all we can ever do is leap into the fray and make better and better mistakes, as none of us is perfect, and human interaction is always fraught with possibilities for disasters and/or triumphs. Mistakes are the ground upon which we stand, and a situation that at one moment may appear to be a mistake could at another moment be viewed as a success or a right action. It all becomes a matter of perspective, positioning, and, of course, experience. The important thing is to have agency and to be willing to act, to be willing to take risks and step out of one's comfort zone in order to learn and to move things forward and become increasingly competent.

Organization of the Book

This book is a culmination of many years of clinical work as a student, a supervisor, a service provider, a site visitor, and a professor. It offers views from multiple perspectives, as well as bits of wisdom gained along the way.

The book is organized to accompany and follow the core competencies and evidence-based practice and practice-based evidence topics that are covered in current practicum seminar textbooks (i.e., Baird & Mollen, 2023; Russell-Chapin et al., 2022). Each chapter ends with questions designed to help students and instructors reflect on some of the issues raised and discuss how they might respond if faced with similar situations.

This book is not a textbook. It is meant to be used as a narrative accompaniment to more traditional internship and practice texts, illustrating and augmenting some of the important learning themes that are covered in these textbooks, and working toward normalizing some of the challenges that students may experience. While only one of my internships was in

DOI: 10.4324/9781003453475-1

psychology, most of my experience has been in clinical social work, and that is an overarching focus of the book. Many of the concepts and experiences can, however, be translated and applied to internships in any of the helping professions.

The chapters are arranged in an order that anticipates many of the issues that interns encounter as they move through the expected developmental phases at their practicum internships and work toward achieving the core competencies outlined by the Council of Social Work Education (CSWE, 2022). These include demonstrating ethical and professional behavior; engaging in diversity and difference in practice; advancing human rights and social, economic, and environmental justice; engaging in practice-informed research and research-informed practice (or "evidence-based best practices"); engaging in policy practice; and engaging with, assessing, intervening with, and evaluating practice with individuals, families, groups, organizations, and communities.

"Signature Pedagogy"

The Council on Social Work Education (CSWE), the national accrediting body for schools of social work, has declared that the practicum internship is the "signature pedagogy" of social work education (2022, p. 20). Practicum internships offer opportunities and experiences that help to develop a foundation from which our professional lives are launched. While we may not have much input into where we are placed, who our supervisors are, or what particular experiences will shape us, we do have the capacity to make the most of the opportunities that we are offered.

Students are often in learning positions of high anxiety as they enter their internships, and it is important to know that we can transform this anxiety into an empowered, highly energized, and exciting pursuit of knowledge and experience. We are paying for these opportunities, and we can make the most of them through an awareness that assuming a position of not knowing, curiosity, openness, and asking lots of questions will most certainly enhance our learning. Flexibility and the ability to be practical and resourceful are necessities as we enter into a wealth of challenging situations in which we must act responsibly and ethically.

Most important is the ability to acknowledge inexperience and seek out the expertise and knowledge of supervisors and colleagues as we embrace a commitment to becoming lifelong learners, always and forever cultivating "beginner's mind". For, "in the beginner's mind there are many possibilities, but in the expert's, there are few" (Suzuki, 2011, p. 21). "Not knowing" is the place where we always want to be (Anderson & Goolishian, 1992). It requires a certain humility and an openness to always be learning new, important, and exciting things. Assuming a defensive "knowing" position interferes with the possibilities of learning new things. We think we know what we will find, and so we end up looking for and discovering only the narrow and limited things that we "know".

A truly open learning position is critically important in this work as we learn from our clients, our supervisors, our colleagues, and our mentors. It is a collaborative position that we will hopefully cultivate throughout our careers, seeking out opportunities to improve our skills and learn new theories and practices to add to our repertoires as the years go along.

A Challenging Landscape

Mirabito (2012) wrote about the ever-evolving challenges that students must face and the need for them to always be developing new skills, as each new generation of students must become prepared to meet the increasingly complicated demands of practice settings. The current landscape includes an emphasis on the natural disasters resulting from climate change, structural racial injustices and inequities, mass shootings, the ongoing impacts of the pandemic (which is becoming an endemic), mental health challenges, substance misuse, the political climate, an unstable economy, and the impacts of the wars in Ukraine and Israel, to name but a few.

Chapters

The following chapters offer lessons that I learned during my four internships: two in undergraduate school in psychology and social work at the University of New Hampshire and two in graduate school at the Smith College School for Social Work. They touch on such fundamental issues as the importance of safety, relationship-building, good (and not-so-good) supervision, the complexities of ethical practice, boundary-setting, suicide assessment and treatment, and professional identity development. I hope that they will offer some entertainment and also some memorable reminders from across the years as you learn from my mistakes and successes.

The first chapter, "Professional Identity", focuses on a discussion of the processes through which a professional identity is attained by acquiring and integrating new knowledge, values, ethics, and such skills as moving from being an unfocused listener to engaging in focused and purposeful active empathic listening. It begins with a look at "imposter syndrome" and offers several stories of the awakenings I experienced during my training.

For example, at the age of 19, while driving a van and picking up clients along the way as I commuted from my hometown to a day treatment program an hour away, I learned to listen differently, assessing for safety and responding to clients where they were, rather than engaging with them in the random mutual conversations I was used to having with most people.

Chapter 2 explores the complexities of ethical practice. It begins with a discussion of the National Association of Social Work Code of Ethics guidelines (National Association of Social Workers, 2021) in regard to the core values of service, social justice, the dignity and worth of persons, the importance of human relationships, integrity, and competence, and gets into some of the difficult and challenging situations I faced as an intern. I offer stories about some of the ethical dilemmas I had to negotiate during my internships, including issues of privacy and confidentiality, conflicts of interest, sexual harassment, and handling incidents that involved violence.

Chapter 3 addresses supervision, a critically important and central part of every internship experience. Good supervision can significantly enhance learning, while supervision that is lacking can significantly impede it. This chapter offers stories of both. One of my early supervisors seemed to be afraid of the clients we were working with and more interested in having me help with her workload and be a companion to her than in teaching me or overseeing my work. I quickly learned to seek out others to learn from in addition to her, which resulted in a rich and diverse experience that served me well in the long run. This is a practice that I would strongly recommend. Many of the clinicians at your internship placements would be happy to grab a cup of coffee with you, consult with you, and answer questions and engage in conversations about their clinical practice.

Chapter 4 looks at safety, an important issue at internships, not only in the office or at the internship site but also during home visits and out in the community. This chapter focuses on the importance of developing awareness, safety strategies, and engaging in self-defense trainings. It offers stories of unsafe situations that occurred during my internships, including an incident of being robbed at gunpoint in Chicago during the second year of my Master of Social Work (MSW) program. Awareness of safety concerns and preparation for adverse situations must be key parts of any internship experience.

Chapter 5 addresses the issue of suicidality. Suicidality is one of the most challenging issues for a new clinician (or any clinician) to face. The enormous feeling of responsibility for assessing each client's safety and for working to help develop hope in another person's life can feel overwhelming. This chapter offers a discussion of how to assess and work with suicidality, along with stories about how I worked with suicidal clients during my internships. These include a story of a client who carried a vial of cyanide with her at all times to reassure herself that she always had "a way out" and a story of a couple who made a suicide pact and followed through with overdosing on their medication together. One of them woke up and "betrayed" the other by calling an ambulance and getting the other to a hospital. Though this ended their relationship, it saved his life, and he went on to have a rich and fruitful life, however compromised it continued to be by the tragic sadness and losses he had experienced.

Chapter 6 addresses the importance of relationship. Never underestimate the power and significance of relationships! Clinical work is all about developing and honoring relationship as the primary vehicle through which change can occur. Interns often underestimate their importance and the importance of the relationships that they develop with clients. This chapter offers stories that illustrate how I learned about the importance of relationships. One story is of a young girl who refused to talk with me during sessions and covered her face with her hands, peeking through her fingers at me from time to time. When I went home for the Christmas break, she made a suicide attempt and left a note for me. She thought that I had left her and wouldn't be back. I hadn't had any idea that I mattered to her at all. In fact, I had thought that she really disliked me and hated meeting with me.

Chapter 7 explores the drawing of boundaries, symbolic lines that delineate separate identities, and paradoxically facilitate the availability of both the clinician and the client to do the work that needs to be done. The importance of drawing clear boundaries is discussed, along with stories of dramatic boundary violations and how they were handled. After one of my internships, I moved to another town, and one of my clients found out where I had moved and followed me there. She proceeded to violate many boundaries, helping me to learn how important they can be.

In Chapter 8 the focus is on endings. All internships begin with an end in sight. Theories and practices of ending are discussed, along with stories of important ending experiences that I was able to have. It can be useful to think about helping people to complete small pieces of work and experience successes, facilitating their development and their experience of positive and satisfying endings. Endings can be fraught with all kinds of feelings, including guilt about abandoning clients, relief that the internship is over, and excitement about successfully completing a piece of work. I ended one of my internships on crutches with a sprained ankle, probably a manifestation of my ambivalence and guilt about having to leave and move along to my next adventure.

1   Professional Identity

Social work is a noble profession, despite the negative reputation that it has often carried in the general public and in the media. With its roots dating back to the early nineteenth century, when upper-class women and men in both church-affiliated and secular charitable organizations worked to address some of the issues of poverty and immigration, social work began as an attempt to help people in poverty learn how to live. "Friendly visitors", volunteers who were women of means and viewed themselves as morally superior to the people they were purportedly trying to help, would make home visits and literally show those in need the "right way" to care for their homes and their children in an attempt to help them to improve their lives and life situations. Such women as Jane Addams and Mary Richmond developed the settlement house and casework models in the late nineteenth century as ways to try to engage those in need in their own transformation processes through the use of community, collaboration, and philanthropy (Reamer, 2022).

Given its origins, rather than being viewed as a profession that is protective and supportive of families, social work has struggled with a negative reputation as a profession that tells people how to live, splitting up families and removing children from their homes. In spite of all of this, many are drawn to the profession because they would like to help others to transform their lives.

The profession has, of course, evolved, growing and changing as theories and best practices evolve over time. Often, people come to the profession having had a positive experience with a social worker who has helped them to change their lives.

Definitions

Professional identity can be defined as "the attitudes, values, knowledge, beliefs and skills shared with others within a professional group" (Adams et al.,, 2006, p. 55). In the profession of social work, professional identity incorporates the values, ethics, knowledge, and skills that supersede the individual identities of a collective group of people who are organized around the

DOI: 10.4324/9781003453475-2

profession's pursuits of service and social justice. The process of professional development consists of the acquisition of knowledge and skills; understanding the profession as it relates with one's individual identities, values, and beliefs; and finally incorporating these into the creation of one's own personal and idiosyncratic professional identity (Tseng, 2011). The development of one's professional identity is made up of accumulated experiences and knowledge as well as socialization processes, and it continues to evolve throughout one's training and career over a lifetime.

Roulston et al. (2018) studied the learning activities that social work interns found most useful as they worked on the development and internalization of a professional identity. Students ranked being given constructive feedback about their progress, thinking critically and reflectively about their role, discussing values and feelings about their practice, learning about policies and procedures, being provided with consistent supervision, discussing and reflecting on practice skills, and being able to observe supervisors and other staff among their top ten activities for the development of practice competence and social work identity (p. 369).

Professional values, ethics, knowledge, and skills are taught in the classroom before we venture out into the field. We are taught core competencies, practice-based evidences, and evidence-based practices, as well as ethical guidelines and tools with which to develop decisions about how we practice. We learn that from the moment that we enter the profession, even as interns in training, our lives are no longer our own. We become public figures who represent the field, and we are immediately expected to assume certain responsibilities as part of our professional identities. We must behave in certain ways in public and in private, and we are mandated reporters if we are witnesses to forms of abuse and/or neglect.

Awareness and Use of Self

One of the most important aspects of acquiring a professional identity is the development of an awareness of self along with an understanding of how to use one's self. We are actors with agency and responsibility, charged with assessing and intervening with clients in highly complex situations. Moving into a learning position can be difficult, as can be cultivating an openness, curiosity, and, most importantly, a sense of critical thinking, as we begin to take on our new identities. Like stage actors, our training is about honing the instrument of the self. Self-awareness and self-knowledge are ever-evolving and critically important to the development of a professional identity.

This awareness and knowledge of self can be developed through the use of process recordings. These are tools employed in supervision to explore how and why we say and do what we do and say, along with the timing of our choices (to be discussed further in Chapter 3). Many programs and agencies also recommend that interns participate in their own therapy as they work to develop their use of self. This work can trigger and stir up all kinds of issues and feelings that will need to be separated out and contained in order for interns to be successful in their training and in their work with clients.

Imposter Syndrome

"Imposter syndrome" (Clance & Imes, 1978; Vitoria, 2020) and "fake it 'til you make it" come to mind as I think about my evolution of self as a professional social worker. This syndrome is characterized by generalized anxiety, lack of self-confidence, and low self-esteem (Maftei et al., 2021, p. 338), all of which strongly accompanied me throughout my practicum internships.

In many ways I was born to be a social worker. I grew up in a service-oriented family. My mother was a school nurse who later became a psychotherapist, and my father was a high school English teacher who was a very good listener and a promoter of young people's development. Both had followings of people who confided in them and turned to them in times of trouble, which ranged from food insecurity, to pregnancy, to suicidality. I vividly remember accompanying my mom when I was very young as she went on home visits delivering food and clothing to those in need.

While entering a service profession felt like a seamlessly natural thing to do, I also felt like an imposter. I would sit with clients and feel amazed that they seemed to "buy it" that I was in the clinician chair, and they were in the client chair. It seemed that at any moment we could switch positions, and they could as easily be helping me. I felt anxious about sitting with people who believed that I could help them and not knowing enough. I doubted myself and had almost no confidence in myself or in my abilities.

It seems that these are almost universal feelings that interns have, and in many ways, it seems important for these feelings to never completely disappear, as they help keep us feeling humble and honest about our capabilities and intentions and open to always learning. As the years have gone along, I have never really lost the feeling of being an imposter. I often sit across from clients marveling at the fact that I get to do this work and that they seem to believe that I know what I am doing.

When I began my first internship, I felt that I was definitely not qualified to do what I was doing, and it took a lot of courage to "fake it" and behave as if I knew how to do what was required of me. Driving a van and picking up clients along the way, from my home to the day treatment program, were a huge responsibility, to say nothing of being able to engage with them in conversations meant to be therapeutic.

Loss of Autonomy and Privacy

One of the drawbacks of developing a professional identity is that one loses a sense of anonymity and privacy. I have joked with my students, saying that the minute they begin an internship their lives are "no longer your own". I tell the story of having a client say that she saw me out running one morning, and my embarrassment as I tried to remember what I was wearing and wondered whether she saw me spit.

This loss of autonomy was taken to an extreme by my MSW program. They had given lip service to having us choose where we wanted to be placed. The program was an intensive one, consisting of three months of classes over three summers (two semesters with five courses in each) and two nine-month full-time internships (five days each week). One of the draws of the program was that we were placed at internship sites all over the country and were assigned "fly-in people" to support us by reading our monthly reports and process recordings and literally flying in to visit us a couple of times each year, or more often if needed, to meet with us.

Before we arrived on campus, we were sent questionnaires and asked to identify three choices of agencies where we wanted to be placed. While most people were given one of their three choices, some got none of their choices. The consequences were major and life-changing. My second-year placement was in Chicago, not one of my choices, and a city where I knew no one. I was required to move to the Midwest and was luckily not married at the time or in a long-term therapy that might have been disrupted (these things were not considered in the placement decision-making process back then, though I am told that they are now).

Let's Make a Deal

During our end-of-year skit, where we let off a little steam and roasted some of the faculty, we performed a take-off of the game show "Let's Make a Deal". The game consisted of contestants being called up to the stage from the audience to bid on unknown treasures hidden behind various curtains. We called different contestants to the stage to bid on their placements. "Suzy Social Worker, come on down!" "Ann Gree, come on down!" They then chose their placements from behind one of three curtains. This was how it felt to be beginning in this program and in this profession. It was a game of chance, and our lives were already not our own.

Diving In

The development of a professional identity takes time and a lot of chutzpah. As mentioned, when I began my first internship, I was 19 years old and had just completed my first year of college. My placement was at a day treatment center, and I drove a van five days a week during the summer months, picking up clients along the way from one rural town to another, staying all day to co-facilitate groups and counsel people, then driving everyone home. This was while waitressing every night from 5 p.m. to 1 a.m. It is hard to believe that I was given such responsibility at such a young age, and that I was able to stay awake and alert enough to take advantage of such a rich opportunity!

I quickly learned to listen and to speak differently as I got to know the clients. My role was to not develop friendships, but to constantly assess for safety, and to maintain boundaries when asked about my life, opinions, beliefs, or advice about things. I was able to gather important information about each of my passengers each morning and to share it when we arrived at the day treatment program during morning rounds, where staff checked in with one another and reported on clients. I quickly became an integral member of the team; colleagues were very supportive of me and my learning, and my input seemed to be valued.

My second internship was on the forensic unit of a state hospital. This was a more formal and anxiety-producing setting. The unit was locked, and each day I had to walk down a corridor lined with men in cells who would rattle the cell bars and make catcalls (a scene that could have been out of the movie *Silence of the Lambs*) as I walked by. The staff seemed unfriendly and maybe a little burned out. This was a very dark place to intern at, and, in many ways, I learned who I did not want to be as I developed my professional identity.

I can remember going onto another locked unit as an intern at the Veteran's Administration (VA) Hospital when I began my third internship, and walking past a line of patients who would try to kiss my ring as I walked by. Many of them had psychotic illnesses and/or had suffered significant traumas in the service, and they were responding to my name, calling me "The Lord". It was funny. And uncomfortable.

In my fourth internship I was placed on an inpatient unit in a large psychiatric hospital and was able to also see clients in their outpatient clinic. I was able to work with several different supervisors (one primary and others who specialized in working with children, older adults, and families). This was a rich learning opportunity for me, with a diverse client population and many excellent learning experiences.

Role Models

A big part of the development of a professional identity has to do with developing a strong sense of self, shared values, and a sense of professional purpose and expectations (Moorhead et al., 2019, p. 983). How does this happen during an internship? I would say that for me, it happened largely through observing role models and picking and choosing mentors who embodied ways of being that I wanted to emulate.

I can remember a psychiatrist at the VA Hospital generously inviting me to sit in with him while he contracted with a client who had a history of violent outbursts in sessions. He began by asking the client to sign a contract with him, saying that he agreed that he would not hit the psychiatrist during the session. The client signed the contract and immediately punched the psychiatrist in the face! The psychiatrist, visibly shaken and with a bright red fist mark on his cheek, said, "I don't think you understood what you just signed". He read the contract to him, had him sign it again, and the client punched him in the face again! I was horrified! I learned that contracts are sometimes not at all useful. He was someone I did not want to emulate.

The doctor who consulted to the drug unit was, however, someone I admired and wanted to learn from. He was able to reduce some very tough men to tears—masterfully, quietly, and respectfully—when he interviewed them during rounds. For many of these men, treatment really began after a session with him. One thing that he would do was to ask them questions about their lives. He would say, "that's bullshit" if he thought someone was trying to get over on him. He would also ask them about their families, particularly about their mothers, and most of them would begin to cry at this point. I learned the importance of family for these men, and I learned that it was important to be real and to question what I didn't think was genuine.

Humor and Irreverence

I also learned from him the importance of irreverence, a strategy that Marsha Linehan has recommended that we use with clients diagnosed with borderline personality disorder (Linehan, 1993), though I believe it is useful with all people. The use of humor, along with irreverently saying things that are unexpected, helps to encourage a human connection when working with all people. It seeks to capture the client's attention with the hope of shifting and widening their perspective and affective responses, helping them to become more available to a relationship that can help them to feel a certain agency and motivation to change. For example, "A client says they're going to kill themselves, and Marsha says, 'Dear, I thought we agreed you weren't going to quit therapy'" (Chapman, 2023). Irony, Humour, and Irreverence | DBT (dbtvancouver.com)

Questions

1. *Reflection.* In your journal, write about your beginning experiences of becoming a social work professional. When did you first become aware that your identity was changing? How was this for you?
2. *Small Group Discussion.* Discuss the ways in which you first experienced your identity beginning to evolve as a social worker. Were you excited? Were there any frustrations or disillusionments that you experienced?
3. *Class Discussion.* What are some of the high points and low points of entering the social work profession?

2 Ethical Practice

Every helping profession has an ethical code that helps to guide its professionals in their decision-making judgments and behaviors as they work with their particular populations in need of services. Of utmost importance is an awareness of the power differential between professionals and those they seek to help, as they interface with people who are, by definition, in a one-down position. The very act of seeking help renders most people into a vulnerable position, and we must work to help them to feel supported and collaborated with when at all possible. Our goal is to help people improve their lives and life circumstances, not to wield power over them.

First, Do No Harm

While interns are often afraid of harming their clients, it is important to know that although we are likely to make many mistakes as we work with people, we really can't hurt them. They won't let us, as their defenses are likely to protect them from harm. The universal code of "first do no harm" that undergirds all healthcare practices is said to have originated from the Hippocratic Oath taken by physicians as they enter their profession, which says to "abstain from doing harm" (Smith, 2013). Most interns are kind and well-meaning people who are in this profession not for the glory or the financial gain, but to help people and to promote social justice, working in whatever ways they can to help make the world a better place.

For the profession of social work, the National Association of Social Work's (NASW's) Code of Ethics (2021) offers clear and complex guidelines that undergird all of social work practice. It spells out the six core social work values of service, social justice, dignity and worth of the person, importance of human relationships, integrity, and competence, and offers principles and standards with which to make decisions when there are ethical dilemmas. Which is often.

The practicum is where the rubber hits the road, so to speak, and where we are able to practice making difficult decisions under close supervision as we work in agencies and other settings with clients who are grappling with

DOI: 10.4324/9781003453475-3

complicated life situations. One of the ironies of ethical practice is that there often really is no one "right" answer to an ethical dilemma. Outside of the mandate to not have sexual relationships with clients, and the mandate to keep people safe if they are being abused or neglected or if they are a danger to themselves or others, many of the dilemmas are complex and engender wide gray areas, leaving a lot of room for discussion and decision-making.

It is important to be able to hash things out with colleagues and with supervisors as we go along, coming to decisions that are well-informed and collaborative. In these complex decision-making situations, it is also important to document the specifics of the ethical dilemmas and to list the people with whom we have collaborated as we come to our decisions about how to proceed.

The first core competency that students must learn is to "demonstrate ethical and professional behavior" (CSWE, 2022, p. 8). Ethical dilemmas pose thorny challenges to all practitioners, especially to trainees who tend to feel disempowered in their learner positions. During my internships, I was faced with several challenging ethical dilemmas: some privacy and confidentiality dilemmas, a conflict-of-interest dilemma, a sexual harassment dilemma, and a dilemma in which a patient prone to violence attempted to physically assault me, as we shall see in the following pages.

Always Ask Questions

Though there are extreme power and responsibility imbalances between interns and their mentors, interns are in a unique position to always ask questions. New eyes and new perspectives offer major learning opportunities for all involved. I was trained to look at situations from as many perspectives as possible, to think critically, and to respectfully challenge ways of doing things. Organizations, systems, and the workers who people them often get stuck doing things in certain ways based on patterns that have been passed along.

An example is the mother who always cut the Christmas roast in a certain way, getting rid of a portion of the roast, and setting it aside. When her daughter asked why she did this, the mother realized that she did it because her mother had always done it. She asked her mother why and learned that it was because when her mother was young, her mother had only had one small roasting pan, and the roast had to be cut that way to fit into the pan! Organizations often develop ways of operating that are passed along without question and may no longer be appropriate or useful. Always ask questions.

Contexts and situations change constantly, and ideally our responses to them come from a "beginner's mind" positioning. Beginner's mind is a state of mind that is cultivated in Zen Buddhism, as it leaves one open to experiencing new things without preconceived notions. "The mind of the beginner is empty, free of the habits of the expert, ready to accept, to doubt, and open to all possibilities" (Suzuki, 2007, p. xiv).

Some of My Experiences With Ethical Dilemmas

Privacy and Confidentiality

Clients are entitled to know that their information and the fact that they are working with us are private and confidential, kept only between them and us. The only times it becomes imperative to violate this ethical code are when there is a situation of abuse and/or neglect, and when there is a danger of self-harm or harming others. In these situations, we are ethically obligated to protect our clients and those they may be harming or planning to harm.

Before I began my second internship, which was at a state hospital, one of my childhood friends told me that her father had been an inpatient there and asked me not to read his records if I came across them. I agreed, and became aware that there might be many possible situations where I happened upon clients that I knew. It is ethically important to opt out of working with people that we know in certain contexts. Of course, in rural communities we will possibly know many people who might seek help from us and/or our organization. It is of utmost importance to evaluate each situation and refer clients that we know well to other clinicians, as appropriate, in order to protect the interests of each client. While it may be fine to work with the person who bags your groceries or pumps your gas, more personal connections need to be respected and protected.

Another confidentiality issue arose when my 21-year-old male VA client began talking quite violently about his collection of guns and what he fantasized he might do with them. He carried a diagnosis of post-traumatic stress disorder, and it was clear that he sometimes dissociated in ways that could become dangerous, given his passionate fantasies and level of anger at certain government institutions and people. After consulting with my supervisor, I decided that I needed to call the police and have them come and remove the guns from his home as a safeguard. I informed him of my concerns, and together he and I were able to call the police and make the request during a session in my office. Had I not been able to get his cooperation in calling the police, I would have needed to violate his confidentiality. Involving him in the process helped to de-escalate the situation and contributed to his feeling of feeling safe, protected, and cared for.

Dual Relationships

Dual relationships are relationships that we may develop with our clients outside of the professional or therapeutic relationship that we have with them. They represent a conflict of interest and are not okay, according to the code of ethics, as they may result in the clinician exploiting the client and using the relationship for their own gain.

For example, a client of mine who was a florist got into a practice of bringing me huge bouquets of flowers and offered to help me out by doing some landscaping and gardening work around the office. While I loved the flowers that he brought and would have loved to have his expert help, it felt exploitative to accept these things, and I had to say, "no thanks", and ask him to stop bringing me flowers. This was difficult, as it hurt his feelings and he felt a bit rejected, but we were able to work through it and maintain the ethical frame that was so important to keeping our relationship safe.

On another note, I once went out to the waiting room to greet a new couple that had been assigned to me. I called their names, and as they walked toward me, I realized that one of them was the doctor who had filled in for my ill gynecologist and performed a pelvic exam on me the week before! In a split second I decided that I could work with the situation, and we continued on our way down the hallway to my office. In that split second, I thought about the fact that I had never met this gynecologist before she filled in for mine, and would likely never see her again in that capacity. I thought about my embarrassment and the importance of not succumbing to the needs of my ego. Above all, it seemed important to meet this couple where they were and respond to their need to engage in treatment with me.

When we got to the office and were seated, I began by acknowledging the situation. I said that I was comfortable proceeding and asked if they were, offering to refer them if they were not comfortable. They said that they were okay with continuing. It was clear that we would not be continuing to have a dual relationship. She had only been filling in for my usual doctor. If the situation ever happened again, we would choose not to go ahead with the exam.

We shared a laugh, said something about what a small world we lived in, and continued with some important and productive work that was perhaps enhanced by the humor of this awkward situation.

Accepting Gifts

The practice of accepting gifts that clients may bring represents a thorny dilemma, as some gifts may be viewed as acceptable while others are clearly not. In determining whether to accept a gift it is important to determine what may be motivating the gift-giving and what impacts accepting or rejecting the gift may have. Consultation and conversation can be extremely helpful when trying to determine whether to accept or reject a gift. While in many cases it may be easier to have a blanket policy that you never accept gifts, things are often much more complicated. Each person must develop their own guidelines for determining how to handle gifts.

When I was an intern placed on an inpatient unit in a hospital in Chicago, most of the doctors and nurses knew that I was a music lover without a lot of money to spare to go to the symphony or to jazz concerts. I would often stop in at my mailbox to find that someone had generously left me tickets to performances that they were unable to attend. It was such a wonderful and uplifting gift to come upon these surprises!

One evening, as I was coming out of a session with a wealthy family, the father pulled me aside to offer me a pair of tickets to box seats at a performance in which one of my favorite singers was starring at the opera house. This was a hard one for me. I thanked him and explained to him that I was unable to accept his gift. I can remember the hurt and surprised look on his face, though he did accept my refusal.

Although the NASW's Code of Ethics does not specifically prohibit accepting gifts from clients, it does caution against taking unfair advantage of a professional relationship, encouraging clinicians to set clear and appropriate boundaries with clients, and avoid conflicts of interest (2021). Had I accepted the tickets, it might have changed our professional relationship, as then I would have felt beholden to the family, and they might have expected me to grant them special favors in my work with them.

Sexual Harassment

Sexual harassment was found, in a recent report, to be experienced by more than 55% of students at their internship placements (Wood & Moylan, 2017), though many of them did not report their experiences. According to this study, about half of those experiencing sexual harassment told no one about their experience, and only 5.6% of those who did talk about it made any kind of formal report through agency or campus mechanisms (Wood & Moylan, 2017, p. 719). The reported reasons included thinking that the incident was not serious enough.

Prior to the advent of Anita Hill and her 1991 sexual harassment case, and the more recent (2017) "Me Too" Movement, I was placed on the Forensic Unit of a state hospital where my male supervisor sexually harassed me. It was hard enough that the patients would rattle the bars of their cells and whistle and taunt me as I walked by. I had begun the year with a female supervisor who transferred me to a male supervisor when she became "too busy" to supervise me. He was relatively young and new to the profession and became interested in dating me. I was uncomfortable and refused, upon which he threatened to fail me if I didn't sleep with him. I told him that I would report him if he didn't stop, and didn't tell anyone about it until 20 years later, when I happened upon him in a professional context (described below).

The Code of Ethics addresses the unethical conduct of colleagues, emphasizing the importance of incidents being reported. I did not report this incident, as I felt it would jeopardize my internship, and I felt extremely vulnerable and embarrassed in this situation. In fact, I never talked about it with anyone until years later, when I was interviewing for a university position and had gotten past the first few hoops to a final interview with faculty and staff. I walked into the room and looked around at the faces of the people there to interview me. There he was! He was sitting there looking uncomfortable, maybe a bit guilty, I thought. I got the job and let my boss and the affirmative action officer at the university know what had happened to me as a student. I told them that I wanted to give him the benefit of the doubt. Maybe he had changed, and I didn't want to ruin his life at this point. I did let them know that I would be willing to come forward if any charges were ever brought against him by another student.

Students are in extremely vulnerable positions, given the imbalance of power between them and their supervisors, agency workers, and professors. It is important, nonetheless, to follow the Code of Ethics and hold all professionals accountable for their behavior regardless of power imbalances. Hopefully, in this day and age, with the advent of the "Me Too Movement", students are able to be supported and respected in their roles and will not fear repercussions if and when they need to report unethical behaviors and practices.

Violence

One morning while the team was going from unit to unit doing rounds at the hospital, I was placed at during my second-year MSW internship, one of the patients grabbed me as I walked by him. I had been taking a martial arts course and quickly used a move to get myself out of his grasp. Though my heart was pounding, I said nothing and just kept walking with the other members of the team. When we got to the nurse's station and they gave their report, I learned that this patient had assaulted one of the nurses during the previous night. I again said nothing out of shyness and difficulty speaking up, or perhaps immobilized by a post-traumatic stress response. This was definitely a violation of an ethical code that required me to inform the treatment team of a patient being a danger to himself or others. While I was just an intern at the time, "just an intern" is not a reason to not uphold the ethics of practice. Our one-down position gives us license to be curious and open, and we are obligated to be ethical and responsible regardless of our status or personality.

Questions

1. *Reflection.* In your journal, write about an ethical dilemma that you have been aware of at your internship placement. What were the competing issues? How was it handled? How might you have handled it differently?
2. *Small Group Discussion.* How would you handle your ethical dilemma in the moment?
3. *Class Discussion.* What ethical dilemma struck you in your small group discussion? Facilitate a conversation about this with the larger class.

3   Supervision

Supervision (or "stupidvision", as we called it) is the vehicle through which interns are able to learn the nitty gritty of the work that they engage in during their internships. It is "the primary method of teaching clinical knowledge and skills and enhancing the development of a professional social work identity" (Miehls et al., 2013, p. 128). Klein (2015) emphasized the importance of supervision around collaboration, teamwork, and learning leadership skills at practicum internships, in addition to supervision around developing clinical skills in working with clients. Important aspects of supervision include mentoring, modeling, supporting, and challenging interns.

Supervisors are legally and ethically responsible for all of the work that interns perform. Supervisors' licenses are literally on the line, and so they must not only teach but must also become aware of pretty much everything that their interns are doing at their placements. They must sign off on their interns' notes and generally oversee every aspect of their work. Through the use of process recordings and structured supervisory meetings two hours each week, I was taught the ins and outs of doing psychotherapy, case management, group work, family therapy, collateral work, and collaborating with relevant community agencies and an interdisciplinary team at each of my placements.

Making Use of Supervision

Interns often have not had any experience with having a supervisor available to them. It is therefore of utmost importance to have a conversation with one's supervisor to determine what supervision is, what the expectations of the agency, the school, the supervisor, and the intern are, to discuss your learning style and to explore how you would like to use supervision and what you would like to get out of supervision. Interns are in vulnerable positions, as their work is being evaluated, even graded. The establishment of a solid and trusting supervisory relationship is an ideal to be cultivated if at all possible.

It is also important for an intern to come prepared for supervision. This is a rare opportunity to get some free and focused guidance and knowledge from

DOI: 10.4324/9781003453475-4

a person who has been in the field for at least several years, has been working at the agency for a while, and is offering their time and expertise just to focus on you and your work and try to meet your individual learning needs. Coming with specific client questions, ethical dilemmas, and questions about particularly challenging situations will help you to get as much as you can from this experience.

There is a fine line between supervision and therapy, as many personal issues may get stirred up in doing this work. As a supervisee you have an opportunity to separate out your issues from those of your clients in supervision, and to learn how to use yourself creatively and effectively to work toward facilitating your clients' growth and development. You may benefit from discussing some of the details of your background and talking about how they may facilitate or interfere with your work with particular clients and their life circumstances. This is not a place to get help with your own personal issues; it is a place to identify and strategize how to handle them if they do get stirred up and interfere with your work.

Many interns (and sometimes supervisors) may dread the supervisory hour(s), and supervision may become an obligatory chore that must be accomplished in order to check off a requirement of internship training. This can become a sad state of affairs, and one to avoid if at all possible. If this is what is happening at your placement, it is important to consult with peers and professors and get some help with making things better if at all possible. The development of a trusting and helpful relationship is optimal, and it is important to acknowledge that this can become a significant mutual relationship that is growth-enhancing for both supervisor and supervisee.

Stressors and Structures

In today's busy world, in which most agencies have long waiting lists, not enough clinicians, and requirements for lots of billable hours, many interns view supervision as something that they have to endure and survive in order to successfully complete their placement requirements and attain their degrees. Many supervisors these days may think of supervision as a burden in their already overburdened schedules, rather than the honor and privilege that it is meant to be.

Supervision can be an oasis for both the supervisor and the supervisee. Offering supervision is a privilege, a marker that one has attained a level of knowledge and skill that has positioned one to become a mentor and a role model for students. It represents a badge of honor, an achievement, and it can be very rewarding and even fun. In order for this to happen supervisors must take their role seriously, making sure to set aside the hours for weekly supervision and to show up and be present for them. Supervisors are there to serve their supervisees, to support them in their work, and to teach and challenge them.

In turn, supervisors' own work can become enhanced, as they bring more energy and awareness to how they are thinking about and sitting with clients, perhaps seeing things more from the perspective of their supervisees. Supervisors are also able to both benefit from the cutting-edge knowledge that their interns bring directly from the classroom. The learning and opportunities can be mutually beneficial for supervisor and supervisee.

The role of a supervisee is to come prepared for supervision and to make use of the time, cultivate a relationship with, and take advantage of the expertise of the supervisor. A learning agreement can help to make sure that interns are able to take advantage of the particular experiences and the hours of supervision that their school requires them to have, breaking things into measurable and achievable goals.

Learning Agreements

Learning agreements spell out the core competencies that students are expected to attain, and the specifics of what students are expected to learn, while clearly delineating the expectations that schools have for agencies and their supervisors. Most programs require two hours each week of supervision time (which may include group supervision or team meetings in which cases are presented and discussed), safety training, as well as a certain number of hours of direct contact with clients, among other things. The learning agreements can be used to make sure that interns and their supervisors are following through on what they have agreed to accomplish within the parameters that they have created together.

Process Recordings

Process recordings are not used as rigorously today as they were when I was training. In graduate school we were required to process every word of every session we had (sometimes as many as 20 each week!). Today, students are required to process one or two sessions each week, if any. Basically, process recordings are a verbatim record (they said, you said) of what happened during a session, complete with observations of nonverbal communication and a cataloguing of the emotions (Karpetis, 2019) that occurred within the intern and were observed to be happening in the client.

They also offer an opportunity to reflect on what you wish you had said, or what you might have said. I consider them to be the primary tool through which students learn to listen carefully, remember what happened, reflect on what happened, and learn to make what I call "better and better mistakes" and think about what they might have done differently. They offer a way to train our brains to carefully observe and recall the intricate details of any interaction.

The supervisor's role is to carefully read each process recording and to offer comments and ask questions about specific choices the intern has made in regard to questions asked, responses made, and actions taken. Process recordings offer a way for the supervisor, without entering the room where the intern is meeting with the client, to get a bird's-eye view of the moment-to-moment interactions that have occurred, along with the intern's reflections on what has happened. This can speed up the process of making "better and better mistakes".

Saying Hello

For example, how does one say hello to a client? From the very first interaction with a client, we are setting the stage for what is to follow. If the first encounter is in the waiting room, do you walk over and shake the client's hand? Do you lead the way or follow the client as you walk down the hallway to your office? Are you smiling and enthusiastic about the meeting, or do you try to maintain a certain neutrality so as to create a safe space for the client to enter into? What are you aware of as you begin to cultivate this significant new relationship?

It is important to not assume that a client will be comfortable shaking your hand (particularly during Covid) and to wait for cues from the client about how to proceed. Some clients may have a history of abuse and be wary of contact. Some may have a germ phobia. Many may need you to appear serious and understated. Friendly neutrality, careful presence, and the use of good listening skills are important ways to proceed.

I once had a client who had interviewed many possible therapists and chose me because, she said, I was not overly enthusiastic or positive about things. She said that positive and friendly people made her feel nauseated. She didn't trust them, and she needed a more neutral person in order to feel safe.

Maeve, What Not to Do as a Supervisor

When I first began my internship at the VA Hospital, I was stationed on the drug unit with my supervisor, Maeve. She had set up a small desk in a corner of her office for me, and we began with a walking orientation to the unit, an orientation to the hospital, to the outpatient clinic, and then to the VA campus in general.

As we walked around the drug unit, I was surprised to see men with panty hose on their heads, pulled down over their faces. There were also men with signs hung around their necks that called them names and spelled out how stupid they were as they had gone AWOL (absent without leave) and used substances again. These, I learned, were considered to be "cutting-edge" treatment tactics aiming to publicly humiliate, shame, and shun these men, making an example of them for others in the milieu so that they might not engage in the same behaviors. I was not sure that these tactics were effective, as every Friday evening as I headed for home, I would see a long line of men that I recognized from the program with their thumbs out, going AWOL for the weekend.

On that first day as we walked out along a path to the inpatient mental health unit where patients were kept on locked wards, I noticed that Maeve kept a wide berth between herself and those we passed. We entered the building, stepped onto an elevator to ride to the fourth floor, and just before the door closed a person stepped on and Maeve quickly stepped off. I rode up to the fourth floor and waited for her to arrive. When she did, out of breath from climbing the stairs, I asked her what had happened. She said that the person who had gotten on was a patient, and she had gotten off because "I'm scared of those people". (Hmmmm. . . .)

Several weeks later, as we were sitting in a supervision meeting in Maeve's office, an alarm went off, and Maeve immediately dove under her desk, which was against the wall that the door to her office was on. I was sitting on a couch directly across from the door. The door loudly swung open, and a man stood there pointing a gun at me. I froze. Luckily, I didn't have to do anything, as people had seen him come into the building and he was quickly apprehended, thrown to the ground, handcuffed, and led away. (Hmmmm. . . . Aren't supervisors supposed to throw themselves on top of their students and risk their lives to protect them?)

Supervision with Maeve tended to be fraught. In many ways I felt that she needed my companionship and wanted me to fill in for her and carry her workload. I learned to branch out to other units, gain other experiences, and get as much supervision as people were willing to offer. I had coffee with many of the staff clinicians and was able to pick their brains and learn a great deal from them. I ended up with an additional three supervisors as I began seeing patients on the mental health unit, the nursing home unit, and the outpatient unit and was supervised by staff there. I was also able to participate in a supervision group every week with the other eight interns placed with me. In those group meetings we were required to make formal presentations of our work with clients and gained an enormous amount of knowledge from each other and from the facilitators who rotated in each week.

I also took advantage of the "captive audience" of clients on the drug unit and completed assessments on each of them. This gave me the opportunity to develop my diagnostic and assessment skills and proved to be fun for the clients as they enjoyed trying to con me, one-upping one another with their tales of woe.

One high point of my internship at the VA was the monthly case consultations we had with "experts" from the area. Each of the interns had the opportunity to present a case to one of the visiting consultants. It was not only a rich opportunity; it was also fun to spend time with people from other MSW programs and to get a sense of people's knowledge and skills.

During internship placements, it is important to be creative, curious, open, and resourceful. Don't be afraid to ask questions. I would advise interns to actively seek out as many people and learning opportunities as possible at their internship sites. As students, you are in optimal positions to ask for help and develop relational networks with as many professionals as you can. Grab a cup of coffee with someone you would like to learn from, and consult with experts in the field. Take advantage of your position.

Critical Thinking

David was a supervisor at a training institute I attended during my internship at the VA. Several of us at the institute were part of a weekly group supervision with him. We met with him in his office, which was a room with a private entrance in his home.

One day I presented a client of mine who was actively suicidal most of the time. I was looking for help with how to work with her. David's response was to get up from his chair, go to his desk, and take out a black-and-white photograph of ice on a river in winter. He showed it to us and then told a story of a chronically suicidal client that he had worked with for many years. This client had been hospitalized many times for active suicidal ideation with intent and a solid plan. After years of struggle with intractable depression and many hospitalizations, the client had brought this photograph in as a gift to give to David. David said that he had looked at the photograph for a long time, then looked up at his client and nodded. His client left the office and killed himself that day.

This prompted a heated discussion about what a clinician's responsibility is in this situation. I was angry and at that moment lost all respect for David. In my mind when a person comes to a clinician and is suicidal, it is the clinician's job to work with that client toward helping him to live, not to die. The very fact that that person has walked into the clinician's office requires the clinician to do everything in his or her power to help to keep that person safe. Depending on the situation, this could include contracting for safety, day-to-day and minute-to-minute planning, and/or hospitalization.

Often, successful suicides happen on impulse when a person is going through a particularly difficult time. Though David's client had been dealing with his depression and desire to kill himself for many years, he was in his office talking about it, which in my mind meant that he wanted help. As I had lost respect for David, it became difficult to get anything out of the supervision group. I no longer felt comfortable or trusted his guidance. To this day, whenever I see David's name come up for a training or supervision/consultation group, I can still feel that anger.

Julie

Julie, my supervisor at my first Bachelor of Social Work (BSW) internship, the day treatment program where I was placed as an undergraduate student, was perhaps the best supervisor I was fortunate enough to have. I had no idea how wonderful she was until I had had other supervisors and was able to look back and compare all of them. Julie was humble, unassuming, generous with her time and knowledge, and extremely supportive of me while encouraging me to dive in and take risks with the clients.

She met with me religiously twice each week and made herself available to me for questions and consultations otherwise as needed. As the day treatment program consisted mostly of group sessions, she taught me about group process and group facilitation, her area of expertise. She was able to observe me in action and to give constant constructive feedback directly after things that were happening. She also set me up with a number of individual clients and encouraged me to try things and experiment with what I had learned in the classroom. She was gentle and affirming while also not pulling any punches when it came to critiquing my work. I learned to make better and better mistakes, and to view my work objectively as a developing and ever-evolving work in progress.

One thing that was very refreshing about Julie was her openness and enthusiasm for learning from me! I was extremely shy, and she encouraged me to come forward and even present my work and newfound knowledge to other staff members in a low-key and non-threatening way during team meetings. While excruciatingly anxiety-provoking, this helped me in so many ways to consolidate what I had learned, to gain in self-confidence, and to learn to present my work to colleagues.

This was an amazing supervision experience to have at my first internship and, as it turned out, a hard act to follow. Much of the style that I developed in later years when I became a supervisor was based on what I had been fortunate enough to experience with Julie.

Questions

1. *Reflection.* In your journal, write about what you look for in a supervisor. What have been some of your experiences of meaningful/useful supervision? What have been some negative experiences?
2. *Small Group Discussion.* How might you work with a supervisor who is not supervising you in useful or meaningful ways?
3. *Class Discussion.* What constitutes good and useful supervision? How might you let a supervisor know that they are not meeting your supervision needs? It might be useful to role-play this.

4 Safety

I have often commented on the irony that beginning student interns are placed in some of the most difficult front-line in-the-trenches settings and are charged with helping their clients grapple with highly complicated issues and situations. All of this is, hopefully, with careful supervision of course. Resources are often scarce, and situations may be dangerous. Our least knowledgeable and most unskilled trainees are in the position of working with our most difficult and challenging populations, while more senior clinicians tend to be able to pick and choose the people they work with, as well as the settings in which they work.

Safety during internships encompasses the safety of student interns as well as the safety of clients/patients and, perhaps, the safety of the university and of the agency, protecting them from potential litigation if anything should go wrong. Little has been written about this topic, and what little has been written documents that students are seldom prepared to address safety issues. Unsafe incidents are seldom reported in social service agencies, especially during internship (Saturno, 2022) placements, as most interns are reluctant to "rock the boat" or "cause trouble" (Faria & Kendra 2007; Shields & Kiser, 2003; Reeser & Wertkin, 2001; Spencer & Munch, 2003; Zelnick et al., 2013).

Over the years, social work education has been required to respond to the ongoing changes and increasing challenges of the populations served by students and the agencies in which students are placed in order to help prepare students for more and more complicated and sometimes dangerous contemporary practice (Mirabito, 2012). As clinicians, we are charged with assessing the safety of our clients in their environments and helping them to find safe places to be if they are at risk in their living, work, or social situations. We are also responsible for assessing their safety in regard to their potential for self-harm and/or harm to others each time that we meet with them.

As social work interns venture into unsafe neighborhoods and deal with volatile situations, they must be prepared to respond in the most proactive and thoughtful ways. Though relatively rare, there have been some incidents in which interns are exposed to very dangerous situations and are called on to act quickly and responsibly. Awareness and vigilance are important as we

DOI: 10.4324/9781003453475-5

enter into the lives and life circumstances of our clients and the agencies and organizations that serve them.

The National Association of Social Workers has developed *Guidelines for Social Work Safety in the Workplace* (NASW, 2013a) that can serve as a resource for social work interns and their supervisors at their placements. These guidelines address such issues as office safety, use of mobile phones, risk assessment for home visits, transporting clients, reporting practices, and the importance of safety training and awareness. An additional guide (NASW, 2013b) offers guidelines on how to handle clients who present with anger and volatile behaviors, suggesting that students remain calm, give clients space, listen carefully, and empathize with their clients' situations. It also suggests that students take precautions in advance if they are anticipating difficult sessions (i.e., meeting in an open area and alerting staff/colleagues and/or bringing another person to a home visit).

Many (not all) practicum internship sites orient students to the safety protocols of the particular setting that they find themselves in as part of their onboarding process, though this may only consist of a handout of phone numbers to call, or a discussion of which incident reports to file after something has happened. Much of what is otherwise discussed occurs in supervision and has to do with such "common sense" things as the student wearing "sensible" shoes and clothing, not wearing dangly earrings or jewelry that can be grabbed, having no sharp objects on your desk, leaving a setting if you feel unsafe (as in a home visit where domestic violence may be occurring or drugs are obviously being used), letting staff know about a potentially difficult session, and leaving the door open at an agency during the session. Some offices have "panic buttons" that can be used in a dangerous situation or codes that can be dialed on the phone to alert others to what is happening so that they can help.

Cultivating client safety may have to do with attempts at making the waiting area feel welcoming and safe with things like comfortable chairs, signage that welcomes certain populations, and a staff presence (i.e., a registration window that is generally visible to other staff and clients, or security officers if there are any on site). In the office or during a home visit, it is important to always have the client sit near the door and to never get in between a client and the door. Locked doors can be comforting and/or terrifying for clients and staff, as they can offer protection from outside intruders and/or feel like being in a prison. Generally, it is suggested that doors remain unlocked and clients be given an easily accessible escape route to use when they feel threatened or feel that they might become threatening. I once had a client storm out of a session because, he later said, he was afraid that he might hit me. I appreciated his leaving and commended him for his ability to maintain control.

Given the current social/political climate in the United States (tensions around mass shootings, racism, gender identity, GLBTQIA+ [gay, lesbian, bisexual, transgender, questioning, intersex, asexual plus] issues, economic insecurities, and the pandemic), many organizations now offer active shooter safety training as well as self-defense and crisis response training to staff and interns on a regular basis. These consist of "experts" (police, martial arts instructors, mental health teams) coming into agencies several times each year to help staff increase their awareness and develop skills to handle and hopefully prevent potentially unsafe situations.

My Experiences (or Lack Thereof) of Safety Training

I don't remember any focus on safety when I began at each of my four internships. At my first undergraduate internship, I began each day driving the day-treatment program's van and was immediately responsible for all of the clients I picked up on the drive from my hometown to the program. I know that the day treatment staff had to know that I had a driver's license, and they must have asked about my driving record. I have no memory at all of any discussion of my safety or of the safety of the clients on the drive. (Yikes!)

The safety training on the forensic unit, my second internship site, could have been more rigorous, as it was in a state hospital and clients were locked up and had been deemed to be "dangerous". Many had extensive histories of having committed violent crimes. I do know, for example, that we were told to run toward the riot when the riot bell rang, though there was no preparation for what to do when we got there. My first master's level internship at the Veteran's Administration Hospital had no comprehensive safety protocol or training program.

The psychiatric hospital, the site of my second MSW internship, located on Chicago's South Side, definitely had policies about not going on home visits, and they offered escorts to walk us to and from the hospital parking lots, as the surrounding neighborhoods were deemed to be not safe. Otherwise, there was no safety training to speak of. I naively thought that home visits were critically important and was very upset about not being able to go on them. I soon learned that caution and awareness of safety were of the utmost importance in this setting. One of my clients had been raped in the elevator of her building and became pregnant at age 10. She was also a witness to many gunshot incidents in her building. Although Chicago was a city in which guns seemed to be quite prevalent, I received no training on how to respond to dangerous situations there.

Holly: Against Our Wills

Holly and I had not known each other very well before we were placed together in Chicago, "against our wills", as we said. Smith had given us the opportunity of "choosing" possible internship placements, and neither of us had chosen to spend our second internship year in the "Windy City". We were not at all familiar with the city, and we were careful to familiarize ourselves with the different neighborhoods and to only venture into those that we had been told were "safe". I ended up living in Lincoln Park, and she lived on the South Side of Chicago, closer to the hospital where we had been placed.

One beautiful October afternoon, we were walking back from the library in my neck of the woods, where we had been working on our theses (we jokingly called them "feces"), to my apartment in Lincoln Park (a "very safe neighborhood" by all accounts), when we were accosted by three tall black men in broad daylight on the Jazz Strip. (A point of interest, perhaps, Holly was Asian, and I was white.) The man in the middle pointed a gun at us and asked for our money, jewelry, and our bags (which only had books and papers in them). I naively said, "that's not a real gun", and he pushed me up against the wall of a building and said, "wanna find out"? We gave them everything we had, including our questionably valuable theses and books, and they let us go.

We ran to my apartment and called the police to report the robbery. After the police came and we had filed our report, we went back with them to where we had been accosted and knocked on doors to ask if anyone had witnessed the incident. I had seen one woman peering out from behind her curtain, and we talked with her, but she said she had not seen anything. A few days later we went down to the police station and tried to identify the three men by looking through files of mugshots. I couldn't identify anyone, and, while some looked familiar, I was reluctant to impact someone's life by choosing falsely. We were later called in to try to identify men in a line-up, but again it seemed impossible.

Holly had a trauma history and ended up dropping out of the program and going home, as this incident stirred up some of her past traumas. I took Karate and accumulated parking tickets as I refused to walk any distance on the streets. I would park my car right in front of whatever building I was going to and come out with a parking ticket that I didn't have the money to pay. When I was ready to leave Chicago in the spring to return to school, I hooked up a U-Haul to my car with out-of-town plates and was driving away when I was arrested and taken to the women's prison for my unpaid parking tickets. The two policemen who pulled me over threatened to strip search me, a practice that was happening a lot in those days. I was held in a cell all day and allowed to make phone calls until I was finally able to get my friends to gather enough money to come down to post bail for me. A pretty traumatic day!

Lesson learned: Always be prepared and aware of the levels of crime in different areas. Some of this preparation is an awareness that no area is truly safe; anything can happen. A self-defense course is a good idea, as is the importance always of self-care. Always park in areas where you won't be ticketed, and pay your parking tickets if/when you are ticketed.

Will

Will was a 14-year-old Black boy with a history of many inpatient admissions for suicidal behaviors, as well as "acting out" in school and running away from home many times. He had had several residential treatment placements by the time I met him on the inpatient unit during my second-year MSW placement in Chicago. He had been bullied in school and sexually and physically abused by his father for many years. His parents had divorced, and his father had moved out when he was 12 years old. His current admission was precipitated by an overdose using his mother's anti-depression medication immediately after having been sexually assaulted by his mother's new boyfriend.

When I first met with Will for a family session with his mother in my office, he walked in, sat in my chair at my desk, picked up a pair of scissors and some paper clips that I had carelessly left on the desk, and pushed the "panic button" that was conveniently located under the desk. I immediately called the front desk to let them know not to respond to the alarm and asked him to put down the scissors and paper clips. He refused. I decided not to engage in a struggle and took off my watch and gave it to him, asking him to keep track of the time during the session. This sideways move seemed to work to alter the power struggle, distracting him while giving him a job to do and maybe a sense of purpose. He appeared quite belligerent throughout the session, however, refusing to participate in any kind of interaction, and it was clear that his mother was not in charge at all. I had been getting some training and supervision in family systems work and tried to engage them in activities designed to change up the energy in the room and offer positive interactions between Will and his mother, between Will and me, and also between his mother and me.

I asked them if they would be willing to try something, and, perhaps out of curiosity, they agreed. I had them both stand opposite each other, and they played a game where they had to stack red plastic cups into a pyramid using only elastics that they had to join together and pull on to create perfect tension to lift the cups onto each other. This required some communication and collaboration, and they seemed to have fun doing it, laughing, and joking with one another. After they successfully created a pyramid, we were able to sit and talk differently, and Will did not seem to be so intent on pushing the boundaries. We were able to keep things safe without the power struggles he had become so used to.

In power struggles it is important to always get out of the way, and give way, offering the client an avenue to save face and get out of the struggle. When taking lifesaving classes, I was taught that when there is a rip tide, it is critical to not fight it. The ocean is a force of nature that needs to be respected; swim sideways. Sideways maneuvers can be powerful and very effective as clients are able to do something different and move along in the interaction, maintaining their composure and perhaps experiencing some successes.

Anne

Anne was a woman in her sixties who had a history of chronic major mental illness and had lived a lifetime of trauma, including early childhood abuse, multiple psychotic breaks and suicidality, many admissions to inpatient settings, and off-and-on homelessness. When I met her during my second-year MSW internship on an inpatient unit in a Chicago hospital, she had been admitted for a suicide attempt and was floridly psychotic. At one point during a session in one of the small interview rooms on the unit, she leapt up out of her chair, screaming her daughter's name, and put her hands around my throat. My heart was pounding as I stood up and said, "I'm scared. Please sit down". She sat down (!), and I immediately picked up the phone and called the crisis team. When I got them on the phone, they asked if any staff were nearby, as they were in another area of the hospital and couldn't respond immediately. I pushed the panic button to ask for help. Some nurses came running and were able to restrain her and help her to calm down.

I was relieved by her immediate response and learned the importance of being real with clients and connecting with and appealing to their humanness. It was amazing to me that she actually sat down when I said I was scared! In a crisis, it is important to remain as calm as possible and to remember to ask for help from those nearby. It was ironic that I called the crisis team rather than asking for help from those immediately available. Perhaps another example of my not wanting to bother people or rock the boat.

Violence

Violence in the workplace is something that is also under-reported, particularly by students at their internships (Tully et al., 1993; Zelnick et al., 2013). It seems that a certain level of denial is needed in order to be able to venture into the helping professions at all. Often tragic and traumatic events will raise awareness, and research will follow (i.e., the many instances of gun violence). In 2009, a social worker was killed in New Hampshire while conducting a home visit for a residential treatment center (https://patch.com/new-hampshire/nashua/veneer-of-safety-chapter-1). In 2011, a social worker was killed at a Boston area group home where she had arrived and was there to take a resident to an appointment (www.coshnetwork.org/fallen-worker-stephanie-moulton-massachusetts).

Between my BSW and MSW programs, I moved to Boston and worked and lived at a halfway house for two years. After I left there to begin my MSW program the person they hired to replace me was murdered by one of the residents. She was 22 years old and had been alone in the house with him over a Christmas vacation. He was 28 and had had no reported history of violence. He called her over to his room ostensibly to give her a Christmas present, and killed her because, he said, he "just didn't like her". Terrifying.

There were several times during my internships when I was faced with violent situations that I had to respond to. While working at the Chicago hospital where I had been placed, I was making rounds with the team one morning (we literally went onto each unit to receive the morning report from the night nurses) and was grabbed by a patient in the hallway as we were parading through the unit. I quickly used one of my new self-defense moves to get away and said nothing. During the report, I learned that this patient had assaulted a staff member the night before. I again said nothing, partly because I tended to be very reticent and didn't want to draw attention to myself, and partly because I didn't want to "cause trouble".

When I was placed on the drug unit at the VA there were several times when fights broke out and staff had to subdue the patients. There was also a time (previously described) when a patient came into the office where I was sitting in supervision; he had a loaded gun and had to be wrestled to the ground by security. Luckily, staff members had seen him come into the building and immediately called for help. On the forensic unit at the state hospital where I was placed, a riot broke out in the cafeteria one day while I was meeting with a patient. A patient had been ironing his pants and threw the hot iron at a guard. Patients began overturning the cafeteria tables and throwing chairs. Fights broke out. I ran in the other direction, though I had been told that we needed to move in and engage. I was not prepared to risk getting hurt.

I had received almost no training on how to handle each of these incidents. I was lucky that I didn't get hurt. Much of what I did was to use my common sense. I tried to avoid situations and get out of the way, disengage, and count on more experienced staff to handle things wherever possible.

The Code of Ethics emphasizes the importance of promoting the general welfare of society, of communicating professionally with colleagues, and of holding colleagues and clients accountable for their actions regardless of their mental health situation. If a situation is unsafe, it is important to report it and do everything you can to make it safe despite the discomfort of rocking the boat and "causing trouble".

Questions

1. *Reflection.* In your journal, write about times when you have felt unsafe at your internship. How did you handle this? How might you have handled it differently?
2. *Small Group Discussion.* Please tell the group about a time when you have felt unsafe at your internship.
3. *Class Discussion.* How might you handle your situation differently if given the chance? How might others handle it?

5   Suicidality

Suicidality is one of the most challenging issues for a new clinician (or, for that matter, any clinician) to face. The enormous feelings of responsibility for another person's life can be overwhelming and extremely anxiety-provoking. It is helpful to remember that we are not in charge of other people's lives; we can only offer help and throw out lifelines, working to delay impulsivity and engender hopefulness if at all possible. Ultimately, if our clients decide to take their lives, they will, and there is nothing we can do to stop them. While they are our clients and asking for our help, we are obligated to do everything we can to try to help keep them safe. We are also not alone in our endeavors with clients; our supervisors are there to consult with, and, while we are interns, they bear the ultimate responsibility for the work that we do.

There are many things that we can learn about suicide assessment and contracting that can help us to position ourselves to offer help to those who ask when they are dealing with suicidal thoughts or impulses or have developed concrete plans (Feldman & Freedentahl, 2006; Osteen et al., 2014; Sanders et al., 2008; Sharpe et al., 2014). The most important is to consult with supervisors and colleagues. This is an issue that must not be handled alone. The Substance Abuse and Mental Health Treatment (SAMHSA) website offers a comprehensive list of resources for clinicians working with suicidal clients (Help Prevent Suicide | SAMHSA). There is also a free and confidential suicide and crisis lifeline (dial the #988) that clinicians and clients can call 24 hours a day, 7 days a week in the United States with live people ready, available, and trained to help those in crisis. This includes those whose crisis has to do with helping those who are in crisis.

Crisis Theory

Crisis theory (Lindemann, 1944) offers a useful frame for understanding how to approach and work with suicidality. Based on the aftermath of a fire at the Cocoanut Grove Nightclub in Boston, Massachusetts, in which there was a stampede to a door that opened inward and 493 people died, Eric Lindemann studied family members' and friends' responses and developed theories and

DOI: 10.4324/9781003453475-6

practices to offer help in coping with this crisis. He observed that people had a definite pattern of responses to the loss of their loved ones. These included somatic symptoms of exhaustion, a sense of unreality and preoccupation with images of the deceased, feelings of guilt, hostility and anger, restlessness and difficulty initiating and/or sustaining organized activity, and dependency on anyone encouraging positive activity.

A crisis is defined as an acute emotional upset that results in disequilibrium and a breakdown in a person's usual coping abilities (Lindemann, 1944). Lindemann recommended that treaters help clients to express their grief, paying attention to under- and over-reactions, helping clients to find new and rewarding patterns of interaction, and helping clients to talk about guilt and review their relationships with the deceased.

The goal of crisis intervention is to restore equilibrium, perhaps using the crisis to attain novel and creatively different ways of coping. Treatment must be immediate and brief. The clinician needs to be active and direct, offering tangible and practical support with an action plan to help the person get through the minutes, hours, and days following the crisis. Positive support systems need to be mobilized, and the goal of the work is symptom reduction. This may include using medication to help with such issues as difficulties with insomnia or sleeping too much, extreme anxiety, and over- or under-eating in the short term. Survivor guilt and a belief that one's life was meaningless were possible responses to the Cocoanut Grove crisis, and suicidality was one of the symptoms that arose.

Each instance of suicidality is a crisis that offers a dramatic signal that something is wrong. The person's equilibrium is "off" for whatever reason, and immediate actions must be taken to help return the person to a state of equilibrium and, hopefully, a feeling of well-being. Many clients are coping with chronic depression along with their suicidal thoughts, and all too often people around them have stopped listening and taking their hopelessness seriously. Many families may become so overwhelmed with their situations that they may want the client dead, or perhaps they have always wanted the client dead and have been abusing them for years.

Conflicting Responses to Suicidality

There is an ongoing debate in the field about how to manage suicidal ideation and intent. Essentially, the debate is between clinicians who try to tightly manage clients' behaviors, contracting for safety and removing potential means of suicide while involving family members in monitoring safety, and others who work to collaborate with clients, offering choices and the freedom to make decisions about their lives (Jobes et al., 2007). At my internships, I was trained to follow a strict protocol of contracting with clients for safety, working with them and their families to remove potential means of suicide, and hospitalizing clients who were not able to contract or work to keep their environments free of potential means of harm.

In my later practice years, as I became more experienced, and as I was being supervised by clinicians who were comfortable with an alternative approach, I tended to work more relationally and collaboratively with clients. I was able to develop a relatively trusting relationship in which I offered a lifeline to them when they were in distress. I essentially recoiled from the "power over" dynamic that I had been trained to develop with clients and did not always trust that the families who had abused and/ or neglected my clients would have their best interests at heart. I gave my clients a lot of room so that they could develop the tools and internal structures needed to handle their suicidal thoughts and impulses safely over time, recognizing that theirs was often a daily struggle, at times minute to minute, that they needed to learn how to live with. Of course, there were times when clients needed to be hospitalized to keep them safe, as they were in too much of a crisis and not able to manage their feelings and impulses safely.

Taylor

Taylor was a young woman in her twenties who was my client during my second MSW internship. She had a history of incest perpetrated by both her father and an older brother, and her family had become inured to her expressions of pain and requests for help. She would literally stand in front of the television while they were watching and cut her wrists, bleeding all over their white (!) carpet. They would respond by telling her to move out of the way so that they could continue watching their program.

There was a railroad track behind her house, and one of the ways that she coped while her brother and/or father raped her (sometimes together) was to dissociate and focus on the sound of the train going by. She had placed a coin on the train tracks, and the train had ridden over it and flattened it. She carried the coin with her always and would hold it to self-soothe when she was feeling particularly dysregulated.

She had developed a practice of going to different railroad tracks around the city and calling me from wherever she was to say that she was going to jump in front of a train. It was nerve-wracking to hear the train rushing by in the background and not have any sense of control over what she might do. When she called me to say that she was going to jump, I would talk with her briefly, asking where she was (she never told me), then I would ask her to go home and call me from there. She would! And we would then develop a plan for her to get through the next several hours and days until her impulses to kill herself subsided. Luckily, they always did. We had developed a contract that she would call me before she did anything to harm herself, and somehow this seemed to work for her.

The fact that I listened and responded to her as though she was in crisis seemed reparative and healing for her. Life and death situations *are* crises each and every time and need to be responded to as such. Our job is to help people to value their lives and learn how to live beyond the crises that disrupt their day-to-day functioning. Taylor and I began to focus on the times in her life when she felt enlivened, as when she was walking in the woods with her dog. She was able to expand on those times, spending more of her day outside. Eventually, she began volunteering at a dog shelter, slowly coming out of her shy and isolated world and interacting tentatively with others at the shelter. Her world began to open up such that more of her time was focused around living and less on survival and self-harm.

Dissociative Identity Disorder (DID)

It wasn't until my seventh month of working with Lisa that I learned that she had seven separate identities. Lisa was in her thirties and was actively suicidal most of the time. She had a horrendous history of complex childhood trauma that included an incestuous relationships with her father, as well as repeated satanic ritual abuse by a neighborhood group led by her father. She was quite high functioning despite (or perhaps because of) her history. She worked in the medical field, and by the time I met her, she had co-authored more than 60 articles with colleagues. This may have been the product of another form of abuse, as she was a very hard worker who tended to carry the bulk of responsibility for the work of writing and researching these articles.

One day she brought in a beautiful painting, and when I asked about it, she very matter-of-factly said that one of her personalities had painted it. She proceeded to tell me about the seven personalities who lived inside of her, each a different age and gender. She described how each had appeared during an especially unbearable traumatic experience in her life, taking over for the person to whom the trauma was happening. The newer personality had access to all of the memories of previous personalities, while the older (or younger) personalities did not.

One of her personalities was particularly suicidal and would steal medication from the hospital where she worked. She would stockpile it and then bring it in to me, asking me for help to get rid of it so that she didn't impulsively use it to overdose. I would take it from her, walk down to the bathroom with her following me, and flush it down the toilet while she watched. Finally, I looked at our dynamic with her and told her I no longer wanted to participate in this process. She needed to stop stealing. We could by-pass the middle phase where she brought her stolen pile of medications to me and I got rid of them. I was there to help her develop and live her life, not to participate in her self-destruction.

She bought a vial of cyanide that she carried in her pocket with her wherever she went. She used it as a touchstone, saying that it made her feel safe and that she had "a way out" if she ever needed it. It did seem to reassure her. She would put it on her television set so that she could see it in the evenings when she watched TV, and she slept with it under her pillow. I saw no reason to struggle with her about this. It seemed to help her to cope and worked to help keep her alive during our time working together. This was, of course, quite a controversial practice, as most clinicians would have seen the cyanide as a dangerous weapon and required that she get rid of it.

My supervisor supported my instinct to not struggle with Lisa about this, and fortunately she never used it. It seemed to help keep her safe during our time working together.

Rather than needing to focus on struggles about her suicidality we were able to focus on widening and growing her life. She began expanding her social circle, learned to opt out of research and writing projects, and eventually got into a relationship with a woman that seemed to be healthy and brought her a great deal of happiness.

Bipolar Disorder

Martha, a divorced mother of three, was in her forties and had been diagnosed with bipolar disorder. In our work together I learned that she also had a significant trauma history and a dissociative identity disorder, and she would find herself in dangerous and difficult situations from time to time. She was a devout Catholic, who attended Mass every morning. One of the situations that she would often find herself in was that she would "come to" in the red-light district of Boston dressed as a prostitute with some strange man on top of her. She would not remember how she had gotten there and would panic and struggle to get away, a battle that resulted in her often being beaten up.

She absolutely hated her life and her illness and was deeply ashamed of the circumstances she would find herself in. The only reason she stayed alive, she said, was that she felt that she had to be as good a mother as she could be to her three children. In fact, she had made a pact with herself that she would stay alive until each of them was out of the house, waiting to kill herself until her youngest son graduated from high school. She spent years buying and wrapping gifts for all three of her children's future birthdays, Christmases, and her anticipated grandchildren's birthdays.

I saw Martha with her children for family therapy in the outpatient clinic where I was interning. Martha religiously attended a day treatment program five days each week. One day she didn't show up, and her case manager went to her house to check on her. She didn't answer the door, and the day treatment program did not pursue the matter further. They somehow considered this to be a sufficient wellness check; I considered it to be negligent.

Later that week I received a call from her daughter, who said that Martha had consumed a can of dry gas that morning and gone down to the bridge in the town square. The police found her climbing onto a bridge railing and getting ready to jump. They got her down from the bridge and took her to the local emergency room. When I arrived there, she was already blind and deaf, and she quickly went into a coma. They intubated her, and I sat with her and her family while they went through the grueling process of deciding to turn off the machines. I sat with them while they turned them off and later attended her funeral. She was the only client I ever lost, and, while I was devastated, I completely understood her choice to end her pain. I continued to meet with her children, helping them (and me) to grieve and mourn the profound loss of their mother.

Twin

Robert was in his thirties and had just lost his twin brother to suicide. He was the most lethally suicidal man that any of us on the inpatient unit had ever met. He felt profoundly responsible for his brother's death, saying that he had been unable to save him. He was suffering from an intractable depression and had to be on suicide watch 24/7 when he was first admitted to the locked unit. He slowly made progress, "fell in love" with another patient (another "twinship"?), and they were both discharged at around the same time. Shortly after their discharge, Robert returned to the unit. He and his partner had had a suicide pact and had both overdosed on their medication. She had more body fat than he did, and woke up, "panicked" and called 911, breaking her pact with Robert. He was taken to a medical facility in a coma, and when he was deemed to be medically stable, he returned to the unit.

In my couple work with them we talked about the importance of entering into depressed and suicidal feelings, getting under the depths of his feelings and making choices about how he then handled them. He eventually was discharged and got a job as a grave digger in a cemetery, which appeared to be well-suited for him. It required hours of strenuous activity, and he would spend his lunch hour climbing into a grave he had dug and lying down and imagining being dead with all of the worms and microscopic life in the soil. He said he found this comforting and soothing, and slowly, over time, he began to feel that he didn't need to act on his suicidal feelings. We were able to turn our focus to developing a richer life.

I learned the importance of disengaging from the struggle of trying to help someone stay alive. This is a field that is rife with pain, conflict, and despair. Our job is to help people with their lives. They will always have the choice to die, and it is critically important to engage with them around activating agency in their lives so that they are able to feel that they have options and can choose life.

Robert, however reluctantly, was able to find solace in working in a grave-yard, and eventually did not struggle daily with suicidal thoughts and impulses. While his world would always be impacted by the loss of his brother and his feelings of having betrayed him by living, he was able to begin to work on living for himself as well as for his brother during the brief time that we worked together. He began venturing out socially and, however ambivalently, was able to let go of some of his feelings of guilt for having lived.

It is critically important in this work to never work harder than your client. It is important to not engage in "push-me-pull-you" tugs of war. One must work to go deeper and hold the space of despair for and with clients. While there will always be feelings of sadness and depression, the immediacy of those feelings can fade into the background along with the impulsivity to act on those feelings. A fuller and richer life can then become the focus of the work, as suicidality becomes less and less of an issue over time.

Questions

1. *Reflection.* Have you ever worked with a suicidal client? In your journal, write about what the experience was like, or imagine what it might be like if you were to work with a suicidal client. What stories resonated for you? What are the key issues you see needing to be addressed in this work?
2. *Small Group Discussion.* Have you ever been faced with working with a suicidal client? If so, how did you handle it? If not, how might you handle such a situation in the moment?
3. *Class Discussion.* What are some of the things that stand out for you when thinking about working with suicidality?

6 Relationship

As a psychodynamically trained social worker, I learned early on that the most important tool that we have to work with is the relationship that we develop with our clients. We are human beings working with human beings, and it is a privilege to be able to do the work we do. In many ways the therapeutic relationship is the most intimate, honest, safe, and transformative relationship that any of us will ever have the opportunity to participate in in our lives. Unlike our relationships with friends or family, the therapeutic relationship is one in which there is, ideally, complete neutrality and the focus is on the client. Our job is to respectfully, with curiosity and openness, honor the dignity of our clients, and invite them into a collaborative position in which we can look together at their lives and their life choices. Transference and countertransference are encouraged and become information that can be used as we work to develop a healing relationship that can facilitate the client's growth and development.

Philip Ringstrom (2014) said that the core issue in any human life is the negotiation of the landscape of relational connection along with the development of the autonomous self. Our relationships form and impact our capacity to connect with others and to develop a healthy self that is able to have agency and function separately from others. All of human interaction involves relationships of some sort, and it follows that change and healing of the self requires a reasonably trusting relationship if it is going to be effective.

Transference and Countertransference

Transference, or the client's thoughts and feelings that are projected onto the clinician based on past relationships, and countertransference (the clinician's responses to the client based on past relationships) are a core and inevitable part of every relationship (including love relationships) and must be encouraged and utilized as an integral part of the therapeutic work (Prasko et al., 2022; Ringstrom, 2014). While transference and countertransference used to be considered to be negative and dysfunctional responses to be avoided in

DOI: 10.4324/9781003453475-7

psychotherapy, they are now considered to be an integral and important part of every relational interaction. They offer critical information about how the client relates and what may get in the way of fulfilling relationships.

It is important to understand and make use of transference and counter-transference responses in this work. Many of these responses may stem from the power differential between client and clinician, as the client is in need and seeking help, and the clinician is the facilitator of that help. Feelings from past relationships tend to get stirred up and can become a useful part of the interaction in both directions as they inform us of what may be happening on deep and perhaps primitive levels.

For example, a mandated client may enter a first session angrily, expecting to be judged and mistreated by the clinician. The clinician, in turn, may be offended by the client's assumptions and find it difficult to maintain a neutral and open position as they begin this relationship. With multiple levels operating at once, the complexities of relational interaction begin.

Relationship Development

One of my supervisors had a hostess-with-the-mostest style, welcoming clients and emphasizing their comfort as she worked with them. She was keenly aware of the power differential between herself and her clients and, in subtle ways, demonstrated her positive regard for them and her wish to learn from them about their lives and about how she could best be of use to them. She used her warmth and enjoyment of people to encourage positive transference responses that facilitated a certain trust and the development of relationships focused on working together to improve their lives. Her belief was that it was important to not colonize her clients' lives and that they knew best what needed to happen. Another supervisor wore flannel shirts and hiking boots and would lean back and put his feet up on the coffee table in the middle of the room, which tended to help his clients to feel connected and at ease, though it did ruffle the feathers of some who needed a more formal presentation.

Both were invested in helping clients to quickly relax and engage in relationships that focused on their agendas and needs. They recognized that most clients who come for help are anxious and perhaps need help with entering into the relationship, learning how to use the relationship, and taking advantage of what we are offering them. Many have never been in a relationship in which the focus is entirely on them, and so they may need help acclimating and learning about the process of talking about themselves and their needs.

That heart-pounding (exciting and terrifying at the same time) moment of a first interaction with a client is an opportunity to practice some of the fake-it-'til-you-make-it skills that we have been reading and talking about. It is important to remember that this relationship is not about us. The client is coming to us asking for help in a moment (probably) of extreme vulnerability. It takes courage to seek out the help of a stranger, and, whether this first encounter is voluntary or mandated, the first meeting sets the stage for all that is to follow. Empathy, compassion, respect, curiosity, and openness are critical. There are so many things to be aware of beyond our own anxiety and self-consciousness.

Beyond assessment/evaluation and determination of good fit, the purpose of the first meeting is to make a connection and sort out the possibility of a second meeting. Who are you? What is happening? Why are you here? Why now? Is there something that I/we can help you with?

Maya—Cultural Diversity

Maya was a 38-year-old single mother of two who had come to the United States from the Philippines in her twenties to escape an abusive marriage and had been sent to the hospital and put on anti-psychotic medications when she described her anxiety to the immigration officers as a feeling that there were "snakes in her stomach". The officers responded to her as "other", unable to empathize with her and step over the language barrier, and she in turn responded with increased anxiety and incoherence.

When I met her at the day treatment program, she had been in and out of psychiatric hospitals and treatment programs many times. It seemed that most of her issues had to do with the complexities of having been "snowed" with too many medications for years and dealing with the side effects of the medications.

She had not had the language to describe her anxiety early on, and this had sent her on a long journey of what became chronic mental illness. Her two children had had to be placed in foster care, she was depressed and lonely, and she was unable to work or to participate in any form of training or education. Our system had failed her, and it was going to be a long road to being able to function on her own and getting her children back.

The process of developing a relationship with her was a difficult one as she had lost trust in most people in the United States. Rightfully so. Our beginning relationship was very tentative, and we proceeded slowly and gently toward a beginning of learning who we were together. I only knew her for a few months and so was not able to experience the years of long-term therapy and relationship development that her recovery would require. Though we only had a few months to work together, we were able to develop enough of a relationship to hopefully help her with future relationships.

Lisa: Never Doubt the Power of Relationship

Lisa was 16 years old when I met her at my second-year internship placement at a hospital in Chicago. She had already lived a lifetime. She lived in "the projects" on the South Side of Chicago and had been raped in an elevator when she was 10. The rape resulted in a pregnancy, and she had had the baby and given him to her mom to raise as her sibling.

She came to see me in the outpatient clinic as she was depressed and struggling with basic functioning. She spoke only minimally and would sit with her hands over her face and peek through her fingers at me from time to time. I mostly just sat with her and focused on my own breathing and tried to put myself in her shoes. Every 15 minutes or so I would say something. I would ask her a question (which she would not answer) or talk about what she might be thinking or feeling. I felt completely inadequate.

I began to ask her to nod if what I said came close to what was happening for her. She began to respond. She would nod when I said things like, "you seem uncomfortable" or "you don't know what to say". She had never been in therapy before, and certainly had no idea about what happened there. I began explaining what was possible and spelling out how things might go.

I suspected that it didn't help that she was black, and I was white and not much older than she was. I was from a small town in the Northeast, and she was from a big city in the Midwest. I asked my supervisor if I could make a home visit to meet her family and get to know her more. She said that I could not venture into her neighborhood; it was way too dangerous, and there were often gang shootings there. I invited her mother and family to come in, and they refused.

And so it went. Fifty minutes each week of silence that was torturous for me and, it seemed, for Lisa. She did show up religiously and didn't appear to have a problem with coming to our sessions. I offered to play board games and card games; Lisa participated wordlessly. This went on from September to mid-December, when I left for a two-week Christmas break.

Upon my return I learned that Lisa had overdosed on her medication and had written a suicide note addressed to me! The note said that she was worried that I had left her and wouldn't return. I was shocked. I had had no idea that I (or the work we were doing together) meant anything to her. Apparently, it had become important and was at the center of her life. I visited her in the hospital (people stayed inpatient for months, even years back then), and we were able to pick up our weekly sessions while she was still on the inpatient unit. She began talking, and things changed dramatically.

When she was discharged, we continued our work in the outpatient clinic. She was able to begin to talk about her life and what had happened to her, and we were able to develop more of a relationship before I unfortunately had to leave and return to school. I transferred her to another social worker before I left to return to campus, and hopefully our relationship helped her to develop a productive relationship with her new therapist.

Never doubt the impact that a consistent, caring, and non-threatening relationship can have. *And*, remember that it is the relationship that matters above all else.

Self-Care and the Relationship With One's Self

It can't be overemphasized that our relationship with ourselves is of paramount importance as we engage in this profession and in this work. We need to know ourselves very well in order to be of use to the people we are working with. We need to know where we leave off and others begin, how we respond to certain issues, and what kinds of things might be triggering and/or overwhelming to work with. We need to be able to say that there are some people that we are not comfortable working with and refer them to others who are able to work with them.

While not required, it is often recommended that students and interns engage in their own personal psychotherapy in order to have a place and person that is theirs, get some support, and learn more about themselves and about how the relationship might feel from the other side of the process. It also can help with separating out some of the triggering issues, and learning strategies to cope with what comes up. Interestingly, I got into therapy while I was in Chicago, and one of my supervisors told me that I really needed to be in an analysis, that therapy would not be enough. I wasn't sure what that meant, but I didn't have the money, the time, or the desire to be in a more intensive therapy. I stuck with what I was doing, and there was a bit of tension with my supervisor after that. In many ways it was important that I draw a line and take care of myself by not following her advice.

It is important to always tend the fire of your presence and connection with your clients by taking good care of yourself. Value them by showing up, being present, and participating with them in genuine interactions. This requires that you always work at developing and learning about yourself. You *and* they will be changed through the vehicle of the relationship and through engaging in the processes of change together.

Questions

1. *Reflection*. In your journal, write about your experiences of developing relationships with clients. What are some of the key issues to think about as you engage in this work?
2. *Small Group Discussion.* What has been your experience of working with clients who have had difficult attachment histories? How have you thought about and worked with these kinds of clients?
3. *Class Discussion.* Please share with the larger group some of your examples of attending to the relationships you have with clients. What have you found to be challenging? What has seemed easy in this work?

7   Boundaries

Boundaries, or lines that clearly delineate where we leave off and others be-gin, are critical necessities in this work. Rather than limiting us, they serve to promote our integrity, or wholeness, and are, paradoxically, able to increase our accessibility and availability to our clients. Ethical practice requires that practitioners establish clear professional boundaries between themselves and their clients (National Association of Social Workers, 2021). These bounda-ries help to establish safety and offer clear guidelines about how to proceed in therapeutic relationships. According to Reamer (2005), "boundary issues involve circumstances in which social workers encounter actual or potential conflicts between their professional duties and their social, sexual, religious or business relationships" (p. 121).

Professional boundaries have to do with such things as not having dual relationships (more than one kind of relationship, prioritizing our profes-sional relationship) with our clients, not touching our clients inappro-priately, not having sex with our clients, not having friendships with our clients, not accepting gifts from our clients, and limiting self-disclosure (Reamer, 2005). We are expected to be there for our clients and to focus with them on improving their lives, not ours, though our lives are often inadvertently improved through our work with our clients. This focus can be difficult for many of our clients, as they are not accustomed to focusing on themselves and many may have difficulty developing trust with someone that they know very little about. It can also feel difficult for an intern to learn how to navigate clients' questions and attempts at developing mutual relationships with us.

In graduate school we were taught to respond to clients' questions by ask-ing them questions about their questions. For example, when asked if I had children, I was taught to ask what it would mean to the client if I did have children and what it would mean if I did not have children. This would often lead to clients feeling frustrated and "talked down to". A simple "yes" or "no" might have worked toward developing more of a sense of respect, mutuality, and beginning trust, quickly shifting the focus to the client and to the work at hand.

DOI: 10.4324/9781003453475-8

Positioning and Collaboration

While boundaries are critically important, it is also important that these boundaries are able to sometimes be flexible and permeable so that we avoid power differentials as much as possible (though they are inherently there by definition between clinician and client) and work relationally human-to-human without exploitation of the relationships that we develop. Clear and strong boundaries can limit opportunities for evolving relationships with our clients; they are also at times necessary to promote safe and careful relationships with our clients.

Combs and Freedman (2020) wrote,

> ...orienting oneself by asking, "Where must I draw and enforce my boundaries?" leads to perceiving a different world than the one we inhabit through asking, "What sort of relationship does this situation call for?" and, "What are the effects of my actions on this relationship and its members?"
>
> (p. 60)

They point out that many of the narrow and rigid boundaries that we have traditionally been required to establish are fear-based, emphasizing the "otherness" of our clients and trying to avoid risk and litigation. While maintaining clear and safe boundaries with their clients, Combs and Freedman emphasize the values of interdependence, collaboration, and community in their work, inviting clinicians to participate in ways that privilege clients' voices and agendas. In this way they work to flexibly ask clients what is important to them and how they can together work to open up a sense of agency in their lives, rather than imposing their limited agendas on them.

The kinds of boundaries that we are required to establish really depend on our development and comfort levels as clinicians, and on the development and comfort levels of our clients. Many internships are set in agencies that offer services to clients with significant poverty, mental health issues, housing issues, substance misuse, family issues, and so on. The clients served by these agencies may tend to need firmer boundaries than those needed by a client who is higher functioning, for example. Their symptoms and life circumstances may predispose them to test boundaries or violate them, as we shall see in the following narratives. Beginning clinicians tend to be more comfortable with firm and inflexible boundaries. It is important to be aware of our shared humanity, however, and, as much as possible, to come forward as we call our clients forward in respectful and boundaried ways.

Curious questions and a relational focus can help to alter the power imbalances that are inherent in this work. Rather than evaluating and "treating" problems and people, curious questions open up an emphasis on collaboratively working to widen awareness and possibilities with them. In order to facilitate this, Combs & Freedman pose such questions as:

> "Whose voice is being privileged in this relationship?" . . . "Is anyone showing signs of being closed down, not fully able to enter into the work?" . . . "What are we doing to foster collaboration?" . . . "Are we asking if and how our actions are useful, and tailoring them in line with the response?" . . . "Is this relationship opening up or closing down the experience of agency for the people who are consulting with us?"
>
> (2020, pp. 62–63)

Self-Disclosure

One of the questions that interns must grapple with is how much of themselves and their lives to disclose in relationships with clients. Many err on the side of never talking about their lives, while others talk too much about themselves and their issues. This may lead to huge imbalances and power differentials. While the work we are doing with clients is about them and their lives, small self-disclosures (i.e., "I do/do not have children") can facilitate relationships and move the work along. Our clients need to develop a sense of us so that they can feel safe enough to do the work that they have come to do. Clients with trauma histories may have more difficulty than others in feeling safe and may be particularly curious about who we are. Carrie was one of these clients.

Carrie

During my first internship at age 19 at the day treatment program, I inadvertently learned a lot about the importance of clear and flexible boundaries as I got to know the clients and responded to their curiosity and questions during our sessions and the less-structured environment of our drives together.

Carrie was a 38-year-old married mother of two young children when I first met her in the driveway outside of her home. She was quite short and round with curly red hair and deep blue eyes. She appeared animated, friendly, and chatty as she climbed the steps into the van. As she was my first pick-up of the day, she sat in the front seat, and we had some time to talk while we drove to the next stop to pick up the next client. I had had a bit of supervision and training prior to this first encounter but felt under-prepared and in over my head with the responsibilities I had been given. She asked many questions about me and my life, and I did my best to respond without talking too much about myself.

She asked me about school, friends, whether I had a boyfriend, my family, what brought me to this work. I answered briefly, trying not to appear to be rude, and asking questions to keep the focus on her and her life. The fact that we were driving and that the situation was informal made it difficult to use the usual deflecting statements like, "we are here to focus on you and your life".

She told me that she had been diagnosed with bipolar disorder and had been hospitalized many times for suicidal ideation and suicide attempts. She said that she had "always wanted to die, more or less" as her life was extremely painful, given her illness. During the manic phases of her illness, she was unable to stop singing 24/7, which, she said, was very painful for her. During the low phases, she could barely move, and spent her time planning complicated suicide attempts.

Throughout the summer we had many long talks, and I became caught up in her cycles of suicidality. I vividly remember her plan to steal the car keys from her husband's jacket pocket, drive out to a remote place in the woods, and overdose on her medications so that no one could find her and revive her. It was difficult for me to be in charge of dropping her off each day, given her palpable pain and her sometimes definite and detailed plans. I learned how to perform suicide assessments and developed daily safety agreements with her. She became very attached to me, and I later learned that she kept tabs on me through information she got from the staff long after I was finished with this summer internship.

After I graduated from college and moved to Boston, the staff, who I had kept in touch with, made the mistake of telling her where I would be working. That fall she also moved to Boston. I was working at a halfway house where I lived in as an overnight staff member. One weekend when I was away, Carrie came to the house and told my colleagues that she was a friend of mine and I had said that she could stay in my room for the weekend. She slept in my bed (Goldilocks), read and wrote in my journal, stole some of my clothes, and left before I returned. I felt violated and angry when I came back and discovered what had happened. I contacted the day treatment staff and also spoke with my current colleagues about the importance of protecting my boundaries. I did not pursue finding out how to contact her, and never heard from her or about her again.

Dan

During my second BSW internship on the forensic unit of a state hospital, my first client, Dan, was a man in his sixties who had murdered his mother when he was younger. Rather than feeling frightened by him, I was curious. He was a small, very pale man who seemed to focus inward as if he wanted to disappear. After hearing his story, I could understand how he came to kill his mother, who had been very abusive to him. She had physically and sexually abused him beginning at a very young age. When he was 15, he said, he had had enough, and he fought back one day, hitting her over the head with a hammer. One of the blows hit her temple, and she died. He had been determined to be not guilty by reason of insanity and had been on the unit for 47 years.

When I was first introduced to him, he appeared quiet, respectful, and quite docile. I met with him for our sessions at a table in the corner of the cafeteria, where we could be closely observed. A guard would bring him out in handcuffs, uncuff him, and stand close by monitoring our sessions, which prevented any physical boundary violations. He didn't ask me any questions about myself and only cooperated in responding to mine about him.

One day, as we were meeting, the riot bell sounded, and all hell broke loose. Men were running through the cafeteria, upending tables, and I can remember one, who had been ironing his clothes, threw a hot iron at another. We had been told to run toward the chaos so that we could help, though not trained as to what to do once we got there. I quickly ran in the other direction and got out of the building, leaving my client there to cope with the chaos and breaking the frame of our meeting. I essentially violated the boundaries of the internship, deciding that I wasn't going to risk my life to follow the protocols of the unit. Luckily, there were no repercussions for this, and perhaps it helped my relationship with Dan.

My work with Dan was to try to break down some of the defenses he had developed over the many years that he had been confined to the locked unit. He had been abused as a child, then bullied and harassed by others on the unit for most of his life. Trust was all but impossible for him. I would like to think that our work offered an experience of a relationship that was respectful and perhaps more positive than those he had been used to. He did open up a bit, though the progress was incremental and our relationship was brief.

Steve: Red Shoes—Compassion, Empathy, and Gullibility

Steve was a young man in his twenties who had landed on the forensic unit repeatedly. He would "do his time", be discharged, and go out and rape young women who, he said, "wanted it". He would be arrested for statutory rape and re-admitted to the forensic unit each time when he was deemed to be not guilty by reason of insanity. When I asked him why he continued this pattern and was so "good at getting caught" (a paradoxical intervention), he said that he had "grown up in the system" and it was all he knew. He said that he was looking for "three square meals and a roof over his head". I had never thought about things in this way. I had never thought that someone would want to be locked in an institution and might think of it as a caring and nurturing home.

One morning I came in to find Steve waiting for me outside my door. He was all dressed up in a suit and tie, though he was still wearing his signature red high-top sneakers. He appeared quite upset, and, although he was not my client, I invited him to come into my office (a boundary violation right there), where he sat and told me that he had just gotten a phone call and learned that his 2-year-old daughter had been diagnosed with leukemia and her prognosis was not good. He said that he had gotten a pass and was on his way to visit her. He appeared genuinely distraught, and my eyes teared up as I sat with him.

When he got up to leave, he came over and hugged me. I was immobilized and didn't know how to stop him at that point, though he was breaking a boundary. I have never been able to figure out how to stop a person from hugging me when they are coming toward me, and the hug is already in motion. I did have a client once who would engage in a dance with me in which he would come toward me, and I would step out of the way as he moved past me. It became our idiosyncratic fun way of ending each session, a symbolic hug.

After we had finished talking, I went down to the office to write a note in his chart and, when I read the chart, I learned that he had fabricated the whole story. He didn't have a daughter! She didn't have leukemia. I felt angry and violated. He had definitely manipulated me and clearly got a kick out of "playing me". I marched down to the locked unit and, amidst the usual catcalls and rattling of the bars, confronted him. His response was to laugh and mock me, preening in front of his fellow inmates. I realized in retrospect how gullible I had been and how foolish it had been for me to invite a person who repeatedly raped young women and who was not even my client into my office unsupervised. I was lucky that more hadn't happened, and I learned the hard way that I needed to be clearer about the boundaries I was setting or not setting.

Many of the men on the forensic unit were not ready to engage in any kind of genuine relationship. They were extremely hardened and guarded, and they seemed to view interactions with me as entertainment rather than something that might have the capacity to help and change them.

Sadly, I learned to listen to everything with some distance and to be a little cynical and suspicious about the truth of some people's stories. It is, intrinsically, so important to believe everything that clients say, though always taking things in with a grain of salt. While knowing that all will not be accurate, there are pieces of truth underneath every interaction, and it becomes fascinating and challenging to sort things out.

Learning the Hard Way

These examples of boundary violations, while not devastating and thankfully not dangerous, were extremely uncomfortable. I learned to be more careful and clear about my boundaries. I learned that with some clients it was important to be quite conservative and a bit rigid with my boundaries, despite the power dynamics that this engendered. Some clients, like Steve and Carrie, who were not at all clear about their own boundaries, required firm and inflexible boundaries. I also learned that I could not count on staff to always have defined boundaries and that the drawing of clear lines had to also extend to them.

While some clients do require firm and inflexible boundaries, others, like Dan, need help with learning how to be flexible and collaborate more mutually. With Dan, our shared humanity seemed more important than the power differential between us. It is important to individualize our work with clients and to think about what sort of relationship each situation may call for.

Questions

1. *Reflection*. In your journal, write about how you handle setting boundaries. Are some boundaries more difficult to set than others? How might you work to establish collaborative relationships with clients?
2. *Small Group Discussion.* Please talk about some challenges and successes that have occurred in your practice of setting boundaries with clients. What have you learned? What might you try to do differently?
3. *Class Discussion.* What are boundaries, and why are they important in clinical work? What has been your experience of setting boundaries with clients?

8   Endings

Endings, or terminations, as they are called in the world of social work and psychology, can be very mixed for all involved (Rosenthal et al., 2007; Siebold, 1991, 2007). As an inevitable and significant part of every clinical relationship, endings can offer powerful vehicles for growth in dealing with issues of separation, loss, and, perhaps, unresolved grief (Aafjes-Van Doorn & Wooldridge, 2018; De Geest & Meganck, 2019). They can also be viewed as opportunities for joy, and a celebration of a job that has been well done, as we look back at what we have accomplished, take measure of where we are now, and look forward to the opportunities for growth in the future.

Internships are, by their very definition, time limited. We begin each relationship with our clients knowing that there is a clear and specific end in sight. Often, agencies assign clients to interns that they believe can handle the fact that the work will be relatively brief. Some agencies have what they call "frequent fliers", who are routinely assigned to interns. These are clients for whom the agency represents a significant lifetime and often an intergenerational relationship. For these clients, the important dependency is on the organization and the stability and services it has to offer, which it has offered to their family for generations over time. The specific clinicians are less important than the organization, which has become a significant part of the family system.

Siebold's (2007) article on "forced termination" offers a look at the importance of relationship as a "core element of the helping process" (p. 91) and delineates some of the positives and negatives of termination for clients and clinicians. Among these, she lists regression, guilt, and abandonment, as well as the opportunity to experience a positive ending.

Regression

"The nature of training in the helping process inevitably brings benefits, but it also frequently repeats the hurtful experiences of the past" (Siebold, 2007, p. 95). Regression, acting out, avoidance, and protest may go hand in hand with the development of an increased ability to tolerate sadness, have a

DOI: 10.4324/9781003453475-9

positive experience of ending, and perhaps experience a feeling of relief during the termination process.

Often, clients who have had negative experiences of endings are able to rework some of their unresolved feelings and issues when they have a planned termination. They may be able to express some of the anger and sadness that they had not been able to express before. Hopefully, they will be able to process feelings that they have not been able to work through related to abandonment or loss from separations and relationship break-ups or even deaths.

During the termination process, many clients (and some clinicians) will fall back into patterns that they have been working to change. Clients may come late or cancel appointments, and symptoms that they brought with them may reoccur or intensify (anxiety, depression, sleep disturbances, substance use), making it difficult to go forward with the termination process. Clinicians may forget things or develop problems once again in completing paperwork, for example. Competence that has been attained may feel impossible to hang onto.

Guilt and Abandonment

Students often feel guilty about needing to end the relationships that they have so carefully cultivated with their clients. They talk about the difficulties of abandoning the people who have histories of abandonment and who have been able to develop a beginning level of trust with them. They may feel that they have exploited their clients in order to further their education, offering them something that can never be delivered. It can be helpful to think about the work they do with these clients as a form of brief treatment. It can also be useful to remember that the energy, focus, new perspective, and enthusiasm that students bring to their work have offered these clients a valuable and useful experience of relationship. Clients may have the potential of experiencing endings that are positive for the first time in their lives and of accomplishing smaller pieces of work successfully. Some clients turn things around and are able to feel proud of having contributed to the education of an intern.

A Form of Brief Treatment

Some clients may not be happy to be working with interns, and they may terminate the work prematurely. Some may terminate early because the "fit" is just not right, or perhaps the scheduling does not work, or they may be concerned that the intern is too young and inexperienced to handle them and their concerns. Hopefully, in these instances, they can be referred to another clinician so that they can complete the work that they came to accomplish.

Miguel Leibovich (1981) wrote about the importance of helping clients to experience "tolerable small successes" (p. 260), a construct I have found useful when working more briefly with clients who have not been able to have positive and constructive connections with people. It is useful to positively frame the work we have been able to do as a solid piece of completed work that the client can feel finished with and satisfied with, if that is at all possible.

Punctuation

The process of termination can be seen as one of punctuation, marking a moment in which we take a breath, look to the past and to the future, and say goodbye to the present. In the case of clinical work, there is always (in my opinion) more therapeutic work to be done, and there will be opportunities to continue the work at another time in the future if the client is interested. Hopefully, the relationships that clients have had with students will offer them beneficial or "good enough" experiences for them to want to continue the work with another therapist if and when there is more work to be done.

Many internship settings have natural termination moments. A project that you have been working on for several months may come to completion or a school year may be coming to an end. For many internships, the interactions are naturally time limited, so terminations or endings are happening all of the time, as are beginnings. For example, in inpatient hospital internships or in hospice settings there are natural time limits, discharges, and deaths that occur as a matter of course.

Marking the Moment

The process of termination includes a review of the work that you and your client have been able to accomplish together, an assessment of what issues might still need to be worked on, and recommendations about where and when and how to proceed.

In their book *Narrative Means to Therapeutic Ends* (1990), Michael White and David Epston (1990) wrote about marking the ending of a piece of work with a diploma that they would create specifically for each person or family that they worked with. On the diploma they would inscribe such things as "Congratulations to _____ for Conquering the Sneaky Wee" for a child who had been struggling with bed-wetting, for example. It is useful to mark an ending with a token of the work you have accomplished together. It can be a simple piece of paper with a listing of the work that has been done or a small object, such as a stone, that the client can carry with them and that may have a lot of meaning to them and remind them of an important relationship and a job that has been well done.

Let the Ending Match the Relationship

Regardless of the time frame, it is important when ending to be sure to honor the relationship and the nature of the work that has been done. It is also important to not overdo endings. The quality and intensity of the termination needs to match the quality and intensity of the relationship. *And* assessment must continue to occur until the final moment. We can never anticipate what might have been stirred up during our interactions and the work we have done together or what might be stirred up through the process of ending.

Rory

Rory was a 35-year-old male Vietnam veteran who had come to outpatient therapy for help in dealing with his post-traumatic stress disorder symptoms. Since his discharge from the army two years prior, he had been having difficulty sleeping, nightmares, flashbacks of "horror scenes" in which he saw his buddies being killed, startle responses to loud noises in crowds, and difficulty managing "a lot of anger" in his relationship with his girlfriend. He lived alone, struggled with maintaining his employment as a construction worker, and tended to drink and use alcohol and marijuana to self-soothe.

We began working together in September, and it took Rory many months to begin to develop some trust with me. Although I had let him know in the beginning of our work together that I would be leaving in May, he had not remembered and appeared to have a strong reaction to the news when I told him in March that we would need to begin working toward ending. He said that he would not have begun working with me had he known that I would be leaving, and he couldn't believe that I was abandoning him like everyone else had been doing all of his life. Though his relationship with his girlfriend was a relatively new relationship, many of his friends and family members had distanced themselves from him, and he described himself as "toxic". He had been starting fights for no reason and having difficulty even being in the same room with most people.

It was not until the last ten minutes of our final session that Rory told me that when he was in the service, he had driven a cargo truck into his own barracks and killed several of his fellow soldiers and friends who had been asleep. He had been court-martialed, imprisoned, and dishonorably discharged. A few years later, he had been arrested and charged with driving drunk and high into oncoming traffic, in what he said was an attempt to kill himself. He was very tearful and ashamed as he told me all of this, and I felt horrified, not only by what he had been carrying but also by his timing in the telling of it. I didn't know what to do! There was no way to handle this in the now five remaining minutes. I was in over my head, and so I told him that I needed to take a minute to consult with my supervisor and went to find her.

This was not his crisis. It was definitely mine at this point. He had been living with this information for many years, and, in effect, this was his way of confessing to me what had happened as we were saying goodbye. Luckily, my supervisor was available and was able to quickly point out these things, shoring me up so that I could go back into the room and finish our work together. I thanked him for telling me about his past and told him that I really appreciated his ability to tell me. I assessed his current suicide risk, which he denied. I had already referred him to my supervisor, and they had had a meeting to begin their work together. He knew that she had been overseeing my work with him for the past several months, and I assured him that I believed he would be in good hands.

We were able to say goodbye in a way that felt safe and okay despite the chaos. It was definitely not my idea of a good ending, but it really did seem to be a window into the world that Rory had been living in. In a way, his telling me was a gift to me and to him. It opened up a definite pathway for his healing to continue with my supervisor and helped me to accept that the work is always ongoing and there are no neat little packages to be tied up and delivered as we move into and out of our clients' lives.

A Multiplicity of Endings

It is important to recognize that interns must say goodbye to not only all of the clients with whom they have been working, helping each of them to bring the work to some closure, but they also must say goodbye to colleagues, supervisors, and agency staff members as well as classmates, faculty, and perhaps even many consecutive years of being a student. All of this can be overwhelming for some, while for others it can feel like a relief. Freedom. For most, it is a mixture of things.

Hopefully, the intensity and the number of endings can help with practicing and honing the skills involved in facilitating the ending process. It is important to recognize how you handle endings and to perhaps become intentional and set goals about improving your abilities and capacities rather than becoming numb or inured to the emotions and processes of ending.

How *do* you handle endings? Are you someone who slips out the back door without acknowledging that you are leaving or saying your goodbyes to people? Do you gloss over endings as if they don't matter? Perhaps because they matter too much?

Many people say that they are not good at saying goodbye. This cannot be an excuse. It certainly does not give you license to gloss over the termination process. The internship setting and experience require that you learn how to become good at saying goodbye. If not for yourself, because you are responsible for facilitating the processes of other people.

A good ending must include a review of the work that has been accomplished, a look at unfinished business, and an identification of future work that might be recommended. An acknowledgment of the relationship that you have developed together is also important, as the capacity to establish meaningful connections will hopefully be carried forward into relationships that will follow.

Ankle

As I was preparing to wrap up my first MSW internship and return to campus for my second summer of coursework, I was feeling excited to be ending, though stressed and anxious about all of the work I had to tie up at the VA while anticipating the move back to campus and all of the work that I would be doing over the summer. One evening I went out for a run, my head full of all of the things that I had to get done, and inadvertently tripped over a tree root, landing sprawled out on the sidewalk. I had twisted my ankle, spraining it badly (luckily not breaking it). I finished out my placement on crutches and needed to elevate my wrapped ankle during sessions. Not a very professional look.

The guys on the Drug Unit had a field day with my situation, teasing me and making fun of my situation, though they helped me in true gentlemanly fashion, opening doors and carrying things for me while I hobbled around.

One of my outpatient clients, who had a history of violence and a large collection of guns that we had had to have the police confiscate, seemed particularly impacted by (shaken by?) my predicament. During our first session with my foot elevated, as we were reviewing all that we had accomplished together, he said, "I could take you right now, you know". (I thought, he could always have taken me, he must be feeling especially vulnerable right now as we are wrapping up our work together.) I just matter-of-factly responded, "Of course you could take me. I just know that you won't", and he didn't.

We had developed a real and trusting relationship in which he was able to feel safe and also kid around, while acknowledging our relationship and all the work we had done around his depression, social anxiety, and guilt about things he had had to do during the war. Although our relationship had been relatively brief (five months), the brevity seemed to have helped make it possible for him to come forward and say and feel some things that he had never been able to say and feel before. We were able to finish our work together in a way that left him open to continuing with someone else if and when he decided to pursue the work at a later date.

Thoughts

As I am coming to the end of the writing of this book, I am aware of the continued awe and privilege that I feel at being able to do this work. Having the license and capacity to enter into intimate and boundaried relationships with so many amazing, resourceful, and resilient human beings is inspiring and so rewarding. I am ever grateful to all of the people whose lives I have touched and whose lives have had such an impact on my life.

Questions

1. *Reflection.* In your journal, write about how you tend to handle endings. What endings have gone well? What endings have not gone so well? Why? What have important transitions or endings taught you about the importance of ending well? What are some of the skills you need to develop to perform the tasks of ending?
2. *Small Group Discussion.* Discuss what you have learned about ending well with clients. Have there been any endings that have surprised you? What skills and tasks are important for ending well with clients?
3. *Class Discussion.* What have you learned about endings with clients? What do you do well in these endings? What do you still need to work on?

References

Aafjes-Van Doorn, K., & Wooldridge, T. (2018). The complexity of loss during a forced termination: A case illustration. *British Journal of Psychotherapy*, *34*(2), 285–299.

Adams, K., Hean, S., Sturgis, P., & Macleod Clark, J. (2006). Investigating the factors influencing professional identity of first-year health and social care students. *Learning in Health and Social Care*, *5*(2), 55–68.

Anderson, H., & Goolishian, H. (1992). The client is the expert: A not-knowing approach to therapy. In S. McNamee & K. J. Gergen (Eds.), *Therapy as social construction* (pp. 25–39). Thousand Oaks, CA: Sage.

Baird, B., & Mollen, D. (2023). *The internship, practicum and field placement handbook*. Abingdon, Oxford: Routledge.

Chapman, A. (2023, August 22). Irony, humour, and irreverence. https://dbtvancouver.com/irony-humour-and-irreverence/

Clance, P. R., & Imes, S. A. (1978). The impostor phenomenon in high achieving women. *Psychotherapy: Theory, Research & Practice*, *15*(3), 241–247.

Combs, G., & Freedman, J. (2020). Relationships, not boundaries. *Journal of Systemic Therapies*, *39*(4), 58–71.

Council on Social Work Education (CSWE). (2022). *Educational policy and accreditation standards*. Alexandria, VA: Author.

Dbtvancouver.com. (n.d.). Irony, humour, and irreverence. Retrieved August 22, 2023 from http://dbtvancouver.com/irony-humour-and-irreverence

De Geest, R. M., & Meganck, R. (2019). How do time limits affect our psychotherapies? A literature review. *Psychologica Belgica*, *59*(1), 206–226.

Erikson, E. (1994). *Identity and the life cycle*. New York: Norton.

Faria, G., & Kendra, M. A. (2007). Safety education: A study of undergraduate social work programs. *The Journal of Baccalaureate Social Work*, *12*(2), 141–153.

Feldman, B. N., & Freedenthal, S. (2006). Social work education in suicide intervention and prevention: An unmet need? *Suicide and Life-Threatening Behavior*, *36*, 467–480.

Help Prevent Suicide | SAMHSA. (2023). www.samhsa.gov/suicide

Jobes, M., Moore, M., & O'Connor, S. (2007). Working with suicidal clients using the collaborative assessment and management of suicidality (CAMS). *Journal of Mental Health Counseling*, *29*(4), 283–300.

Karpetis, G. (2019). In-depth learning in field education: Evaluating the effectiveness of process recording. *Journal of Social Work Practice*, *33*(1), 95–107.

Klein, E. (2015). Supervision of social work interns as members of a multidisciplinary team. *Research on Social Work Practice*, *25*(6), 697–701.

Leibovich, M. (1981). Short-term psychotherapy for the borderline personality disorder. *Psychotherapy and Psychosomatics*, *35*, 257–264.

Lindemann, E. (1944). Symptomatology and management of acute grief. *The American Journal of Psychiatry*, *151*(6), 155–160.

Linehan, M. M. (1993). *Cognitive behavioral therapy of borderline personality disorder*. New York, NY: Guilford.

Maftei, A., Dumitriu, A., & Holman, A. (2021). "They will discover I'm a fraud": The imposter syndrome among psychology students. *Studia Psychologica*, *63*(4), 337–351.

Miehls, D., Everett, J., Segal, C., & du Bois, C. (2013). MSW students' views of supervision: Factors contributing to satisfactory field experiences. *Clinical Supervisor*, *32*(1), 128–146.

Mirabito, D. M. (2012). Educating a new generation of social workers: Challenges and skills needed for contemporary agency-based practice. *Clinical Social Work Journal*, *40*(2), 245–254.

Moorhead, B., Bell, K., Jones-Mutton, T., Boetto, H., & Bailey, R. (2019). Preparation for practice: Embedding the development of professional identity within social work curriculum. *Social Work Education*, *38*(8), 983–995.

National Association of Social Workers. (2013a). Guidelines for social worker safety in the workplace. *NASW*. Retrieved from www.socialworkers.org/practice/naswstandards/safetystandards2013.pdf

National Association of Social Workers. (2013b). Managing clients who present with anger. *NASW*. Retrieved from www.socialworkers.org/assets/secured/documents/practice/managingangerinclients.pdf

National Association of Social Workers. (2021). NASW code of ethics. Retrieved April 12, 2022 from www.socialworkers.org/About/Ethics/Code-of-Ethics/Code-of-Ethics

Osteen, P., Jacobson, J., & Sharpe, T. (2014). Suicide prevention in social work education: How prepared are social work students? *Journal of Social Work Education*, *50*(2), 349–364.

Prasko, J., Ociskova, M., Vanek, J., Burkauskas, J., Slepecky, M., Bite, I., Krone, I., Sollar, T., & Juskiene, A. (2022). Managing transference and countertransference in cognitive behavioral supervision: Theoretical frame and clinical application. *Psychology Research & Behavior Management*, *15*, 2129–2155.

Reamer, F. G. (2005). Boundary issues in social work: Managing dual relationships. *Social Work*, *48*(1), 121–133.

Reamer, F. G. (2022). *The philosophical foundations of social work*. New York, NY: Columbia University Press.

Reeser, L. C., & Wertkin, R. A. (2001). Safety training in social work education: A national survey. *Journal of Teaching in Social Work*, *21*(1–2), 95–113.

Ringstrom, P. (2014). *A relational psychoanalytic approach to couples psychotherapy*. New York, NY: Routledge.

Rosenthal Gelman, C., Fernandez, P., Hausman, N., Miller, S., &Weiner, M. (2007). Challenging endings: First year interns' experiences with premature termination and discussion points for supervisory guidance. *Clinical Social Work Journal, 35*(2).

Roulston, A., Cleak, H., & Vreugdenhil, A. (2018). Promoting readiness to practice: Which learning activities promote competence and professional identity for student social workers during practice learning? *Journal of Social Work Education, 54*(2), 364–378.

Russell-Chapin, L., Sherman, N., Chapin, T., & Ivey, A. (2022). *Your supervised practicum and internship*. Abingdon, Oxford: Routledge.

Sanders, S., Jacobson, J., & Ting, L. (2008). Preparing for the inevitable: Training social workers to cope with client suicide. *Journal of Teaching in Social Work, 28*(1–2), 1–18.

Saturno, S. (2022). Violent crime and social worker safety. Retrieved from www.socialworktoday.com/archive/exc_032511.shtml

Sharpe, T., Frey, J., & Osteen, P. (2014). Perspectives and appropriateness of suicide gatekeeper training for MSW students. *Social Work in Mental Health, 12*, 117–131.

Shields, G., & Kiser, J. (2003). Violence and aggression directed toward human service workers: An exploratory study. *Families in Society, 84*, 13–20.

Siebold, C. (1991). Termination: When the therapist leaves. *Clinical Social Work Journal, 19*(2), 191–204.

Siebold, C. (2007). Every time we say goodbye: Forced termination revisited-A commentary. *Clinical Social Work Journal, 35*, 91–95.

Smith, C. M. (2013) Origin and uses of primum non nocere—Above all, do no harm! *Journal of Clinical Pharmacology, 45*(4).

Spencer, P. C., & Munch, S. (2003). Client violence toward social workers: The role of management in community mental health programs. *Social Work, 48*, 532–544.

Suzuki, S. (2007). *Zen mind, beginners' mind*. Boston/London: Shambhala Press.

Tseng, M. T. (2011). Ethos of the day—challenges and opportunities in twenty-first social work education. Social Work Education, 30(4), 367–380.

Tully, C., Kropf, N., & Price, J. (1993). Is field a hard hat area? A study of violence in field placements. *Journal of Social Work Education, 29*(2), 191–199.

Vitoria, A. D. (2020). Experiential supervision: Healing imposter phenomenon from the inside out. *The Clinical Supervisor, 40*(2), 200–217.

White, M., & Epston, D. (1990). *Narrative means to therapeutic ends*. New York, NY: W.W. Norton.

Wood, L., & Moylan, C. (2017). "No one talked about it": Social work field placements and sexual harassment. *Journal of Social Work Education, 53*(4), 714–726.

Zelnick, J. R., Slayter, E., Flanzbaum, B., Ginty Butler, N., Domingo, B.. Perlstein, J., & Trust, C. (2013). Part of the job? Workplace violence in Massachusetts social service agencies. *Health and Social Work, 38*(2), 75–85.

Index

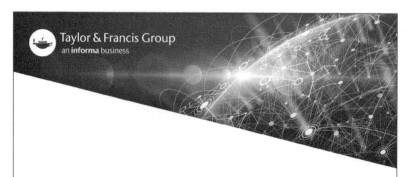